I0039354

LIVE and THRIVE

with

DIABETES

Your Guide to Understanding,
Managing, & Embracing
a Healthier Life

CHRISTINE SCHAFFER
PHARM.D., CPH.

Live and Thrive with Diabetes

Christine Schaffer, Pharm.D., CPH.

Copyright © 2024 Dr. Christine V. Schaffer

All rights reserved. No part of this publication may be reproduced, distributed, or transmitted in any form or by any means, or stored in a database or retrieval system, without the prior written permission of the publisher. Optimal Life, OL, are registered trademarks for the use of their respective owners.

ISBN: 979-8-9900143-1-2

Optimal Life Publishing

christineschaffer.com

Printed in the United States of America

For Worldwide Distribution

A Note to the Reader

Disclaimer: The content within this book is designed for informational and educational purposes exclusively. It should not be viewed as a substitute for professional medical advice. We strongly advise consulting your healthcare provider to thoroughly discuss and evaluate all information and recommendations provided herein, ensuring the formulation of a tailored plan that suits your individual needs.

Dedication

This book is dedicated to my son, Charles, who developed type 1 diabetes in 2004. He has never allowed his diabetes to be an excuse for not accomplishing his dreams and goals. Charles has traveled abroad extensively, is active in sports and mountain climbing, and finished medical school. He has given his family the gift of encouragement, telling us all that individually we can do anything if we really want to. I once said to Charles, "Don't worry. Diabetes doesn't define who you are. You're the same person except that you just happen to have diabetes. Nothing has changed." Charles truly lives life to the fullest.

Acknowledgments

I would like to express my heartfelt gratitude to Dr. Mazin Boushakra for his invaluable assistance in ensuring that the content of this book on diabetes is meticulously updated and supported by the latest references. His expertise and dedication have been instrumental in enhancing the quality and accuracy of this work. Thank you, Dr. Boushakra.

I extend my sincerest appreciation to Aspirex Productions, LLC, and their exceptional team for their unwavering dedication and support throughout the entire process of editing and publishing this book. Their professionalism, expertise, and commitment to excellence have played a pivotal role in bringing this project to fruition. I am immensely grateful to Aspirex Productions for their invaluable contributions and for keeping this endeavor on track with precision and care.

How to Use this Book

Live and Thrive with Diabetes is meant to enhance your knowledge of Diabetes Mellitus (DM) so that you can more fully understand why you need to take control of your diabetes and how to do it. There are three main types of diabetes: type 1, type 2, and gestational. Please note only type 1 and type 2 are discussed in this book.

A summary of the information in each chapter can be found in the Summary and Action Plan Section following each chapter. These sections highlight main facts and review the associated Action Plan.

TABLE OF CONTENTS

Introduction

There are times in our lives when we feel we finally made it. It was a Saturday and I was reflecting where I was in my life. I accomplished my educational goals of receiving a Doctor of Pharmacy Degree in Clinical Science. My national healthcare company was doing well. I was married and had two wonderful children. Best of all, my position at work allowed me the luxury to dive deep into continuing to educate myself on medical and pharmaceutical knowledge. With this freedom to gain all this medical knowledge, I shared it with patients and with healthcare workers, hoping to make a difference in people's lives. It was so satisfying to help people. I especially dove deep into diabetes because it was becoming such an epidemic and I so wanted to help in this area. My disease management company was saving lives and really helping people with chronic diseases to get control instead of having the disease control them.

It all seemed so logical to me. If I could give people the education they needed, then they could use that knowledge to gain control. Knowledge is power, correct?

Then one day everything changed for me and how my disease management company worked with patients. I was in my kitchen cooking dinner while waiting for my husband and son to come home from the movies. They walked into the kitchen and sat down on the stools by the counter. My husband looked at me and said, "Something is wrong with our son." I said, "He is perfect." He replied again, "No. No. Something is wrong with our son." I asked, "Why are you saying that?" He replied, "He kept drinking his huge coke in the movies and went to the bathroom like five times. That's not normal."

Thinking I always have the answers, I told him I had some glucometers and would test his blood sugar. Being the loving wife I was, I said to my husband, "I will test you first. This way I will know that the glucometer is working."

His glucose/blood sugar was just fine. Now I said to my son Charles, "I am going to test your blood sugar." He replied, "OK, Mom." His blood sugar was over 300 mg/dl. Anything equal or over 126 mg/dl is considered to be diagnostic for diabetes. I noticed that he was losing weight, but he had just started track and I thought he was getting in shape. Thinking that the glucometer was not working correctly and to prove it, I grabbed my husband's hand again and stuck his finger so hard, he yelled OW!!! The second test result on my husband was good again. I, the one who understood diabetes so well, started to go into panic mode. So, what do you think I did? I stuck my son's finger again. In my mind I was saying, "This is my baby. Nothing can be wrong with him. HE is perfect." His blood sugar was now over 330 mg/dl.

I was sick to my stomach. I then immediately knew that my son had type 1 diabetes; an auto immune disease in which you develop antibodies to your own cells. His body was producing antibodies killing the beta cells on his pancreas that secrete insulin, creating high blood sugar. I was so upset, but I stood on hope, believing we would overcome this.

Off we went to the hospital before he passed out. I was face-to-face with a disease state that I educated people on and now it was happening to me. As a person with firsthand experience, I now understood the emotions that come from having your disease, in my case, diabetes, control you and your life. We were minutes from my son going into a coma. I held onto my anchor of hope. My son still had a bright future to fulfill.

I wanted answers on what I could do right now to help my son. I wanted to have those answers at my fingertips and know what to do next. I told my son when he was first diagnosed, "Diabetes cannot stop you from accomplishing your goals. You are still the same person; you just happen to have diabetes."

My son was 14 years old when he was diagnosed with type 1 diabetes, and I am happy to let you know that he learned quickly how to gain control of his diabetes. He has since then graduated from medical school and went on to also get a master's in business.

The secret to my son's success was that he learned to control his diabetes and not let his diabetes control him. Yes, there are always challenges, but when you have the right knowledge to know what to do you will be a victor and in control of whatever your chronic disease is.

My son's diagnosis and the lack of easily accessible information prompted me to write self-help chronic disease books. I wanted to make sure that those books included the most important questions to ask your physician and what the answers should be.

My passion for helping people goes beyond words. Living through this experience has made me want to make information on diabetes less complicated, starting with this book. And above all, I want people who have diabetes to know they can control it. It begins with knowledge. Don't let diabetes define who you are. Diabetes cannot stop you from accomplishing your goals. You are still the same person; you just happen to have diabetes.

I encourage you to read through this book. I know if you apply the principles laid out in this book, you will have a better understanding of diabetes, and you will know what is expected of you to gain control over diabetes.

Chapter 1

What Is Diabetes?

My goal for this book is that you live your life and do all the things you want to do because your diabetes is in control. It's time to take back your life and direct it the way you want to direct it. No longer will diabetes control you. You will now control your diabetes.

Understanding how the glucose can get high in the body is the first step in controlling diabetes. Chapters one and two give you the fundamentals that help you build the foundation of knowledge to control your diabetes. Knowledge is power when it comes to health and that is exactly what this book is going to give you. You will not only have knowledge about diabetes, but you will have essential action steps to take and questions in the back of the book to ask your physician. I have also provided answers to those questions which are backed up by the American Diabetes Association. You will no longer feel helpless.

Diabetes is a condition in which there is a buildup of sugar called glucose in your bloodstream. When the glucose gets too high, it has the potential to cause complications in the body that can be very serious. That is why the body works hard at keeping the blood glucose at normal levels.

The two key players in diabetes are **glucose and insulin**. Glucose is a sugar that supplies energy for all your body's functions. You need a constant supply of it throughout the day and night. There are two main ways your body obtains glucose: from the food you eat, and from your liver. During the day your body's energy needs come from the glucose in the food you eat. Any excess glucose from food goes to your liver and is stored in a form called glycogen, which can be released later as glucose when your body needs it. Our body and brain need a constant supply of energy to exist. The liver supplies glucose to our body when we are not getting energy from food. The liver releases small amounts of glucose throughout the day to make sure our body has enough energy. The liver releases the greatest amount of glucose when we sleep because our energy needs are not being met by eating during this time. Insulin is the great communicator. Insulin is a hormone produced in an organ called the pancreas that works with many systems in the body and also regulates the amount of glucose in the bloodstream. Insulin has two important functions:

1. To allow glucose to enter cells so it can be used for energy

2. To regulate the storage and release of glucose in the liver

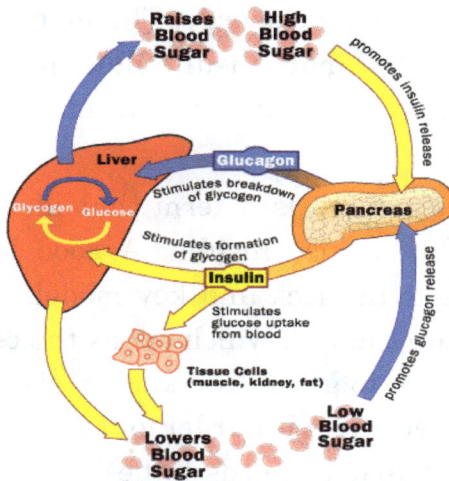

The relationship of glucose and insulin

Diabetes mellitus (DM) is a disease state in which glucose accumulates in the bloodstream. The medical term for this buildup of glucose is **hyperglycemia.** There are two main ways that glucose can enter your bloodstream:

1. from the food you eat,
2. and glucose production by the liver.

When you eat, glucose from the food is absorbed, and insulin is released by your pancreas which is an organ located below the stomach. Insulin is a hormone that allows glucose to go into a cell so it can be used for energy or stored for later use. At the same time, it also directs the liver to slow the production of glucose when the body is getting glucose through food. Think of insulin as a key that opens the door to the cell which allows the glucose to go in. Without insulin, glucose cannot enter the cell; therefore, it builds up in the bloodstream and cells become starved for energy. The more glucose there is in your blood, the more insulin must be secreted from the pancreas in order to facilitate the entrance of glucose into the cell for energy.

Insulin resistance is a term that identifies a cell's decreased ability to use insulin. A good illustration of this resistance is the lock and key model. Insulin is the key that fits into the lock which opens the cell's door and allows the glucose to go in. In insulin resistance, the lock becomes distorted and it is harder for the insulin key to fit. Therefore, more insulin needs to be secreted to increase the chance for some of the insulin to fit in the lock.

As insulin resistance increases, the body compensates by telling the pancreas to secrete more insulin. Over time, the pancreas cannot keep up with the body's insulin needs, and the quantity of insulin released actually decreases as the pancreas wears out. As the available insulin decreases, it has less effect on the glucose from the foods you eat or the liver's glucose production, and glucose levels continue to rise. Eventually, the over worked pancreatic cells that secrete insulin begin to fail entirely, and insulin production eventually stops altogether.

Understanding Diabetes:
Understanding Type 1 and Type 2

Both type 1 and type 2 diabetes result in high glucose levels in your blood, but the origin of how this happens is very different between the two types, and different factors are involved.

Type 1 Diabetes

Type 1 diabetes is characterized by the pancreas being unable to make and failing to secrete insulin. This occurs when the body produces antibodies that kill special cells on the pancreas called beta cells that make and secrete insulin. When your body makes antibodies that kill off the body's own cells it is called an autoimmune response. This response is not normal because the body's immune defenses are meant to kill harmful substances such as bacteria, but not our own cells. The exact role of genetics versus environmental factors in the development of antibodies in type 1 is not known, and currently, there is no definitive evidence that tells us what triggers and causes type 1 diabetes. We do not know if or to what degree environmental factors play a role, along with any genetic factors that may predispose people to the disease.

Because individuals with type 1 diabetes can no longer produce insulin, cells become starved because glucose cannot get into the cells. The body then begins to burn fat for energy, and as a result, individuals with type 1 diabetes are often slender, and upon diagnosis they are usually very thin, with symptoms of urinating a lot called polyuria, extreme thirst called polydipsia, and elevated hunger called polyphagia.

Of all the people who have diabetes, only about 5 to 10 percent have type 1. Type 1 usually develops early in life, and the diagnosis is quick because of the sudden or severe symptoms. However, the autoimmune destruction of beta cells can develop later in life and it is estimated that 5 to 10 percent of people with type 1 develop it after 30 years of age. Overall, the risk for developing type 1 is relatively low. If a parent has type 1, the risk of developing the disease is between 3 and 4 percent and 5 and 15 percent if a brother or sister has type 1. Looking at these statistics, you can see that many individuals with type 1 diabetes mellitus (DM) do not have a first-degree relative (mother or father) with this disorder. There are also certain areas of the world that have a greater population with type 1. Geographically, Scandinavia (Finland, Sweden, Norway, Denmark) has the greatest incidence of the disease. The United States and Northern Europe have an intermediate rate, and the Pacific Rim (Japan and China, for example) has a much lower incidence.[1]

Type 2 Diabetes

Type 2 diabetes has a strong genetic factor. If both parents have type 2 diabetes, the risk factor is 50 percent that it will be inherited by their children. Beyond genetics, type 2 is also associated with environmental or lifestyle factors, such as obesity, lack of physical activity, and poor nutrition habits. Other factors include not enough insulin being secreted by the pancreas, insulin resistance, and increased glucose production, mostly by the liver. Individuals with type 2 diabetes are usually overweight since one of the major causes of insulin resistance is excess body weight. The more excess weight an individual with type 2 diabetes carries, the greater the degree of insulin resistance.

Type 2 diabetes accounts for 90 to 95 percent of people with diabetes mellitus. It is typically diagnosed in older adults, but is becoming more common in younger adults and children as obesity touches an ever-younger population.

Category	Type I	Type II
Age	Onset early in life	Increased onset with age
Prevalence in Diabetes Population	5-10%	90-95%
Cause	Pancreas does not have the ability to secrete insulin. Beta cells destroyed by antibodies.	Not enough insulin secreted, insulin resistance, and poorly controlled liver glucose production
Geographic Location	Highest in Scandinavia, medium in U.S.A., low in Japan and China	Highest in Pacific Islands, intermediate in India and U.S.A. and lowest in Russia
Genetic Factor	Less related to 1st degree relative genetics	More related to 1st degree relative genetics

From Centers for Disease Control

Certain ethnic groups are at a higher risk of developing diabetes than other groups. In 2022, the Centers for Disease Control (CDC) estimated the prevalence of type 2 diabetes in the United States for individuals over the age of 18 as follows:

American Indian or Alaska Native 16.0%

Asian, non-Hispanic	9.2%
Black, non-Hispanic	12.5%
Hispanic, overall	10.3%
White, non-Hispanic	8.5%

Source: Centers for Disease Control and Prevention. National Diabetes Statistics Report website. https://www.cdc.gov/diabetes/data/statistics-report/index.html. Accessed [10/22/2022].

Why is it important to know about diabetes?

Because one hundred years ago people who were born with diabetes eventually starved to death. Diabetes was totally and uniformly lethal. It was not until 1921 that insulin was discovered by Sir Frederick G. Banting and Charles H. Best in a lab at the University of Toronto. How much difference could a century of medical advancements make? The discovery of insulin was one of the greatest medical breakthroughs in history.

The good news is, with the advances of medicine and new drugs, people with diabetes can now live an optimal life when they learn how to be in control. This book helps you to do this.

Today we have the advantage of many medical studies and new medications that help to decrease the complications that have plagued people with diabetes throughout history. This literature tells us that the best strategy is one that is multi-focused on controlling blood glucose, blood pressure, cholesterol and protein in the urine, as well as patient education, diet, exercise, and frequent monitoring to prevent complications.

These same medical studies provide information on how complications can be prevented or slowed down. A person with diabetes does not have to be one of the statistics below.

People with diabetes face the possibility of many complications:

- A two to four-fold increase in risk for coronary heart disease. Coronary disease is the leading cause of death in people with diabetes over the age of 35.

- Diabetes is the eighth leading cause of death overall.

- Diabetes is the leading cause of chronic kidney disease and failure according to the May 15, 2024 National Diabetes Statistics Report. The National Library of Medicine (NIH) reported that 35.6% of people with diabetes had chronic kidney disease.

- Nerve damage, called peripheral sensory neuropathy, may affect up to 50% of people with type 2 diabetes.

- Diabetes is the leading cause of new blindness among adults 20 to 74 years of age.

- Diabetes causes greater than 60% of all non-traumatic amputations.

- 80% of adults with diabetes have hypertension.

- People with diabetes risk increased severity of infections.

- The risk of stroke is two to four times higher than people without diabetes.

When glucose is not controlled, the nature of diabetes is to progress to the complications listed above.

It is my firm belief that education about the disease is the first line of defense in understanding the reasons why these complications may develop and how to prevent them.

Many of us have daily routines in life and it is unlikely that we will change those routines unless we are given a strong enough reason to do so. At the same time, very few of us will intentionally put ourselves in a harmful situation if we actually know of the harm in advance. For example, you probably have a route to work that you drive every day. Imagine that one day, while driving on your usual route, you encountered a big sign indicating a detour because part of the road was washed out in a winter storm. You would take the detour to work.

The detour protected you by giving you important information and you arrived safely at your destination.

But what if you decided to go to work several hours earlier, before the detour was put in place? You would have no prior knowledge that the road was washed out or that you needed to change your route to work. Your normal path to the office has now put you in danger because you had no information that would cause you to do anything differently.

This book is a road map for people with diabetes, showing you the hazards of continuing in the same old way and helping you identify the beneficial detours that will deliver you safely into good health. I want to put as much knowledge as possible in your hands so that you can work intelligently with your physician and other care providers to take charge of your diabetes and keep it in control.

This chapter begins the learning process by explaining what diabetes is, how to control it, what the potential complications are, and how to prevent and control those complications. Each chapter will build on previous information so as not to overwhelm you with a lot of facts all at once, and will start with an introduction and a brief summary to refresh your memory, followed by in-depth information on the subjects discussed.

Diagnosing Diabetes

The classic symptoms of diabetes are polyuria (excessive urination), polydipsia (excessive thirst), polyphagia (excessive hunger), and unexplained weight loss. If you have these symptoms, your physician will probably order the following tests:

1. A fasting blood glucose test

Fasting is defined as no food or drink (except water) for at least eight hours prior to your blood draw. Your blood is then tested for the amount of glucose in it. Your fasting blood glucose results should be below 126 mg/dl (milligrams per deciliter). If your results are 126 mg/dl or greater you should have the test repeated on a separate day to confirm a positive test for diabetes. There are situations where the clinical observation of the patient is so classic for diabetes such as being hungry, thirsty, and urinating all the time, the physician may want to have a random blood glucose drawn to see the results. If a random blood glucose is 200 mg/dl or greater a diagnosis of diabetes can be given.

2. Another test to diagnose diabetes is a two-hour plasma glucose post glucose challenge test (also called an oral glucose tolerance test or OGTT).

In this test you are given a 75-gram glucose drink and your blood glucose is tested two hours later. The test is considered positive for diabetes if the results are 200 mg/dl or greater. This test should also be repeated for confirmation.

3. There is a third blood test to indicate if you have diabetes and it is called Hemoglobin A1C.

Your red blood cells contain hemoglobin, a protein in red blood cells that carries oxygen. When the blood has a lot of glucose in the blood stream, the hemoglobin gets sugar attached onto it. When sugar in the blood is high the sugar spontaneously bonds with hemoglobin. The A1C test measures the percentage of hemoglobin proteins that have glucose attached onto it. An A1C of $\geq$ 6.5% is diagnostic of diabetes.

4. The fourth blood test is a random blood glucose test. Random Plasma Glucose (RPG) is usually done in people with classic symptoms of hyperglycemia.

If glucose levels are 200 mg/dl or greater this is diagnostic for diabetes.

In summary, there are four ways to test and diagnose diabetes.

1. Fasting blood glucose (FPG)
2. Oral Glucose Tolerance Test (OGTT)
3. Hemoglobin A1C (Hgb A1C)
4. Random Plasma Glucose (RPG)

	Normal	Pre-Diabetes	Diabetes
A1C	≤ 5.6%	> 5.7-6.4%	≥ 6.5%
FPG	≤ 99 mg/dL	100 -125 mg/dL	≥ 126 mg/dL
OGTT	<139 mg/dL	≥140-199 mg/dL	> 200mg/dL
RPG			> 200mg/dL

Figure 1.3 Criteria for the diagnosis of diabetes from American Diabetes Association, 2022

A1C, Hemoglobin A1C (hemoglobin that is chemically linked to a sugar). The test should be performed in a laboratory using a method that is NGSP (National Glycohemoglobin Standardization Program) certified and standardized to the DCCT (Diabetes Control and Complications Trial) assay

FPG, Fasting Plasma Glucose. Fasting is defined as no caloric intake for at least 8 hours.*

OGTT, Oral Glucose Tolerance Test. Plasma glucose 2 hours after using a glucose load containing the equivalent of 75g anhydrous glucose dissolved in water.*

RPG, Random Plasma Glucose. Usually done in a patient with classic symptoms of hyperglycemia or hyperglycemic crisis.

In the absence of unequivocal hyperglycemia, diagnosis requires **two** abnormal test results from two separate test samples.

In trying to diagnose individuals who may get type 2 diabetes, it is necessary to define intermediate grades of glucose intolerance. The purpose of this is to identify people who are starting to develop type 2 diabetes, but perhaps do not meet all the criteria listed above, such as a fasting blood glucose greater than 126 mg/dl.

Two terms to be aware of are:

1. Impaired Fasting Glucose (IFG)

Impaired Fasting Glucose is a condition in which fasting blood glucose levels are elevated above what is considered normal, but are not high enough to be diagnosed as diabetes.

2. Impaired Glucose Tolerance (IGT).

Impaired glucose tolerance is determined using the Oral Glucose Tolerance Test (OGTT). The OGGT is performed using a drink that contains a specific amount of glucose. Blood samples are taken at intervals for two hours after drinking the glucose to measure the amount of glucose present in the blood. If glucose levels are above normal, but not high enough to be at diabetes range the individual is said to have impaired glucose tolerance. Either of these conditions signals what is now called **pre-diabetes.**

People who have Impaired Fasting Glucose (IFG) or Impaired Glucose Tolerance (IGT) have an increased risk of diabetes and heart disease. A normal fasting blood glucose result should be less than 100 mg/dl. IFG is diagnosed when the result is greater or equal to 100 mg/dl but less than 126 mg/dl. The following chart sets out the ranges for all these conditions.

Categories of Glucose Tolerance < means less than or equal to < means less than > means greater than or equal to mmol/l means millimoles per liter		
	Fasting Plasma Glucose	Two Hours Post Glucose Load
Normal	Less than 100 mg/dl	Less than 140 mg/dl
Impaired Fasting Glucose (IFG)	> 100 to < 126 mg/dl (> 5.6 to <7.0 mmol/l)	
Impaired Glucose Tolerance (IGT)		> 140 to <199 mg/dl (> 7.8 to <11.1 mmol/l)
Diabetes	>126 mg/dl (>7.0 mmol/l)	> 200 mg/dl (> 11.1 mmol/l)

From American Diabetes Association

Insulin and Insulin Resistance

As mentioned before, insulin is the great communicator that lets your body know if you are fed or starving. Its signals tell the body what functions are needed to survive in either state. Insulin communicates either directly or indirectly with the liver, kidneys, skeletal muscles, adipose (fat) tissues, and with other enzymes throughout your body. Without insulin you cannot survive.

Insulin has many interconnected functions in the body that form a delicate balance between insulin functioning correctly or incorrectly. This balance begins with the amount of insulin secreted relative to the amount of glucose in the blood.

Whenever you are not eating, your liver produces most of the glucose your body requires to continue its activities.

In adults who do *not* have diabetes or insulin resistance, eating a meal triggers the release of insulin. Because glucose is now entering your body from food, glucose from the liver is no longer necessary. Remember, there are two ways glucose gets into the bloodstream; one is from food, and the other is from the liver which produces glucose. Insulin being the great communicator in your body, when it is released in the bloodstream as a result from food, it tells the liver to slow down or stop its glucose production. The body's energy needs are being met by food. The liver can stop producing glucose. Insulin will now concentrate on the body's cells using the key and lock method to open the door of the cells for glucose to enter so it can be used for energy or stored later for use.

Just as insulin helps to decrease glucose in the blood, it also helps the blood stream to have less bad cholesterol. Here is how this happens. When insulin is released, it signals an enzyme called lipase to stop the breakdown of fat cells for energy because, again, energy is being provided by the food being eaten. We do not need fat broken down for energy. This is important because fat cell breakdown results in free fatty acids (FFAs) being released into the bloodstream, which decreases the signaling efficacy of insulin.

Insulin also signals the liver to break down a protein called APOB (Apolipoprotein B). The APOB protein attaches to the bad cholesterol called LDL proteins, and one of its functions is to carry LDL cholesterol into the bloodstream, which is not desirable.

As a review, the major importance of insulin working correctly is:

1. Insulin helps glucose get into the cells for energy, thus decreasing glucose in the bloodstream.

2. Insulin signals the liver to stop releasing glucose when we have energy being supplied by food.

3. Insulin helps to decrease the breakdown of fat cells which results in Free Fatty Acids (FFA). Too much Free Fatty Acids causes insulin to not work well.

4. Insulin helps to decrease the APOB protein in the liver. APOB is a carrier protein that carries the bad cholesterol LDL into the blood stream.

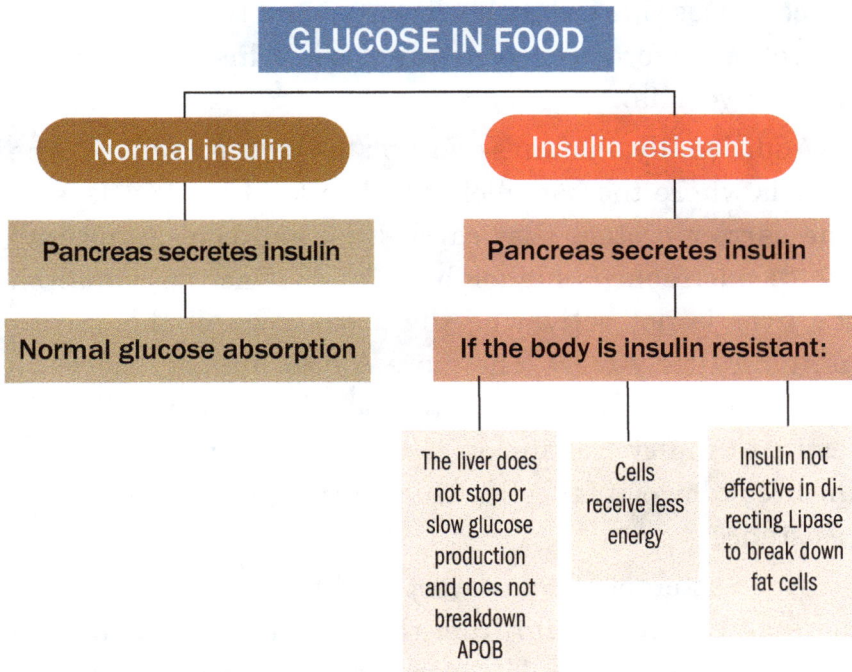

GLUCOSE IN FOOD

Normal insulin

Pancreas secretes insulin

Normal glucose absorption

Insulin resistant

Pancreas secretes insulin

If the body is insulin resistant:

The liver does not stop or slow glucose production and does not breakdown APOB

Cells receive less energy

Insulin not effective in directing Lipase to break down fat cells

It is a different story for people with diabetes and insulin resistance. In insulin resistant individuals, when eating a meal, insulin is released by the pancreas and delivered to the liver where it <u>should</u> suppress the liver's glucose output.

However, because the person is insulin resistant, the insulin is not as effective as it should be, and the liver does not get the message to stop producing glucose and instead continues glucose production. There are two sources of glucose in the body; one from the liver, and another from the food being eaten. Insulin efficacy for getting glucose into the body's cells is also decreased because the key, which is the insulin, is having a hard time getting into the lock on the cell to allow the glucose in. Insulin resistance causes this lock to be distorted and the key not to fit as well as before. The result is marked high blood sugar (hyperglycemia).

Additionally, insulin's effect on the liver is reduced. The liver is where the bad cholesterol called LDL is released. The carrier protein that carries the bad cholesterol into the bloodstream is higher because the insulin signal on the liver is not activating the breakdown of the carrier protein called APOB. The more APOB protein, the more bad cholesterol is carried to the bloodstream. To add insult to injury, insulin is also not effective in stopping the breakdown of fat cells, which further increases insulin resistance.

In an attempt to counteract this, the body will demand more and more insulin from the pancreas to try to keep glucose at proper levels. Over time, the beta cells in the pancreas that secrete insulin become overworked from producing extra insulin on a continual basis and eventually burn out; little or no insulin will be produced. When this finally happens, the individual will become dependent on insulin medication.

But what causes insulin resistance in the first place? Sometimes, it can be a genetic defect in the insulin receptors that causes insulin to be less effective. More commonly, insulin resistance results from a combination of the following factors:

1. Not being able to adequately process the amount of glucose ingested in the food you eat. The cells in your body become resistant to the insulin because of the high glucose.

2. Excessive insulin secretion, which can result in decreasing the availability of insulin receptors needed for insulin to work.

3. Being overweight, which results in more free fatty acids in the circulation, which can interfere with insulin signaling.

4. Lack of exercise, which contributes to weight gain, further increasing insulin resistance.

Our muscles use the most glucose. Approximately 80 percent of total body glucose uptake occurs in skeletal muscle. Therefore, the primary site of insulin resistance in people with type 2 diabetes is in muscle tissue.

Being overweight and having large stores of visceral fat is directly related to insulin resistance. This is because more fat cells create more free fatty acids (FFA) that enter the bloodstream and interfere with insulin signaling. The term **visceral fat or visceral adipose** tissue refers to fat cells situated around your organs, such as your heart, lungs, intestines, liver, kidneys, pancreas, and spleen. This type of fat is different than subcutaneous fat which is stored near the surface of the skin. It is important to distinguish visceral fat from other body fat because **visceral fat has been shown to have a higher rate of fat breakdown than subcutaneous fat, resulting in increased free fatty acid production.** Free fatty acids interfere with insulin's signaling ability and decrease the ability of insulin to allow glucose into the cells, so an increased amount of glucose in the bloodstream is not desirable. Visceral adipose tissue represents approximately 20 percent of fat in men and approximately 6 percent of fat in women.

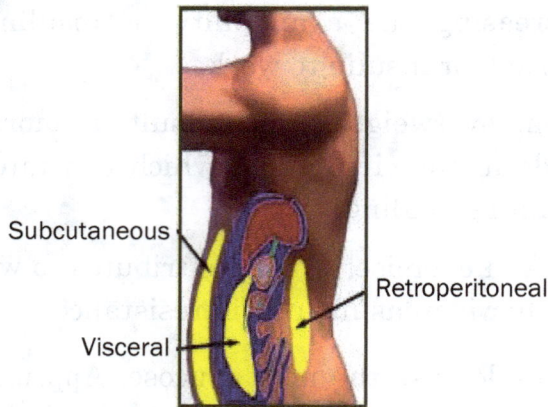

Types and location of adipose tissue

In addition to increased levels of FFAs, type 2 and obese non-diabetic individuals have increased stores of triglycerides in their muscles and liver, and the increased fat content correlates closely with the presence of insulin resistance in these tissues. There is a strong link between insulin resistance and being overweight or obese, and visceral fat is strongly linked to insulin resistance.

In summary, insulin resistance can be a vicious cycle in which decreased sensitivity to insulin causes increased levels of glucose in the bloodstream. The increased demand for insulin production overtaxes the pancreas, which cannot keep up with the body's demand. Over time, it produces less and less insulin, glucose levels continue to rise, and eventually the pancreas burns out and makes little or no insulin at all.

As you can see, being overweight is a strong contributor to insulin resistance and also puts excess stress on your heart, kidneys, and contributes to high blood pressure. Exercise and good eating habits with portion control are a good start to turning around insulin resistance. Working with your physician on the different types of exercise you can do, as well as meeting with a nutritionist to learn about weight loss is essential. When you meet with your doctor, have your blood glucose evaluated to see if you need medication, or if any changes need to be made to medications you are already taking.

Hyperglycemia

The buildup of glucose in the bloodstream is known as **hyperglycemia**. Early signs of hyperglycemia include three classic symptoms:

- **Polyphagia** – feeling hungry all the time
- **Polyuria** – frequent urination
- **Polydipsia** – increased thirst

Other symptoms may include headaches, difficulty concentrating, blurred vision, fatigue, and unintentional weight loss.

Excessive hunger called **polyphagia** stems from the fact that a person with diabetes cannot utilize glucose well as an energy source. Glucose is circulating in the bloodstream, but cells cannot absorb it to use as fuel because insulin is either ineffective or not present in adequate amounts to allow the entry of glucose into cells. To overcome this, the body will attempt to acquire more and more glucose from food, which results in feeling hungry all the time.

Urinating a lot called **polyuria** develops because excess glucose molecules in the blood go into the kidneys creating an effect that pulls water into the kidneys, increasing urine output. As a result, a person with diabetes will need to urinate frequently.

Because a person with high glucose in the blood urinates frequently, they will also experience an increase in thirst called **polydipsia** and desire to drink more in order to replace the fluid being lost in the urine.

These symptoms are more prevalent in individuals with type 1 diabetes, and are less likely to manifest in people with type 2 diabetes. What is important to realize is that if you develop any of these symptoms, you should perform a glucose test right away or talk to your physician to see if your glucose is high, and if so, take action to bring your glucose level down. Failing to do so could require urgent medical attention.

Physical Activity for People with Diabetes

Exercise in people with diabetes has many benefits, such as:

- lower blood glucose concentrations during and after exercise

- lower insulin concentrations

- improved insulin sensitivity

- lower glucose levels

- lower cholesterol levels

- improved blood pressure

- It also helps you lose or maintain your weight, and is great for conditioning your heart.

The American Diabetes Association suggests that adults over 18 years of age perform moderate intensity physical activity for 150 minutes (2 ½ hours) a week, or vigorous aerobic intensity for 75 minutes (1 hour 15 minutes) a week, or an equivalent combination of the two. The guidelines also suggest that muscle-strengthening activities two or more days a week are beneficial.

To maximize an exercise program and make it safe and enjoyable, it is important to get a complete physical exam that carefully screens for the presence of any complications that may be worsened by an exercise program. Your physician may identify times that you should not exercise. For example, if you have type 1 diabetes or insulin dependent type 2 diabetes and your blood glucose levels are above 250 mg/dl (greater than 14 mmol/c) and ketones are present in your urine, then you would be advised not to exercise. Additionally, there are differences in exercise management for people with type 1 versus type 2 diabetes, and your physician should provide you with an action plan on how to manage your diabetes before, during, and after exercise.

Exercise and Insulin

Exercise and Type 1 Diabetes

In type 1 diabetes the hormonal changes noted above are essentially lost because the only insulin in the body is the insulin provided through injection. Once insulin is injected, the amount injected does not change until it is used. With injected insulin, the insulin concentration in the blood stays the same, and the effect may increase if you exercise within one hour following an injection. The absorption of insulin during exercise is increased, especially when the insulin is given immediately before or within a few minutes of exercising. This could lower your glucose too much.

Exercise changes glucose levels by burning off more glucose because glucose is used up when your muscles are more active during a workout. Also, your muscles right after a workout are recovering after a strenuous workout therefore continue to use glucose until recovery is complete. So, if you take insulin and then exercise, glucose utilization and sensitivity are increased, which can lead to hypoglycemia. As a result, the amount of insulin you need is usually reduced. Remember once you take insulin, it cannot be decreased in your body. It not only increases the amount of glucose going into your muscles, but continues to decrease the liver production of glucose, which makes you more susceptible to hypoglycemia. The presence of the insulin and increased insulin sensitivity also decreases the liver's ability to produce glucose, and this can lead to further low blood sugar during long exercise periods. For a long and intense duration of exercise, the body will need to be fed to keep blood sugar from falling too low.

Because of this, everyone with diabetes should have a pre-exercise checklist. Part of this checklist should be an action plan that you have discussed with your physician on the length and exertion level of your exercise program.

Example: Pre-Exercise Checklist for People with Type 1

1. How long should I exercise today?

   If you plan to work out longer than 30 minutes, you may need a snack containing 20 to 25 grams of carbohydrates every 30 minutes. You can determine whether or not you need to do this by testing your glucose during exercise.

   The amount of carbohydrates you may need to consume will vary depending on the intensity and duration of exercise, your level of physical conditioning, what your pre-exercise blood sugar was, and how much insulin is in your system.

2. At what time will I exercise today: before a meal or after a meal? *(Answer: after a meal)*

3. Will my insulin injection be close to when I exercise, and should the amount of insulin be decreased?

4. Check that you have your self-monitoring blood glucose test kit with you and several test strips. Check your blood glucose before, during, and after exercising!

5. Work with your physician to develop a blood glucose level action plan for exercise. Here is an example:

If blood glucose is less than 100 mg/dl, eat a pre-exercise snack.

If blood glucose is less than 100 – 250 mg/dl, no snack is needed.

If blood glucose is over 250 mg/dl, check urine ketones. If positive, do not exercise until ketones are negative.

6. Always carry snacks and water when you exercise.

Post-Exercise Glucose Levels

So, now you have your pre-exercise checklist that your physician has approved, and you have just had a great day of skiing or playing basketball. You are relaxing in your favorite chair, watching a great movie, and your blood sugar goes low, or really low. What just happened? You did all the right things!

You may have stopped exercising, but your muscles are still active, requiring nutrients. Also, increased insulin sensitivity may persist for several hours, and can last for up to 24 hours. This is because of three mechanisms:

1) insulin sensitivity lasts longer, meaning more glucose than normal is being delivered to your muscles;

2) because of the increased insulin sensitivity, the liver is producing less glucose; and

3) the liver's glycogen stores are low due to your recent exercise.

Because everyone reacts differently to exercise and requires varying amounts of glucose, only experience with your exercise program and observing how your body responds will provide the answer to the question posed above. Therefore, the more you test your blood glucose after exercising, the more you will understand your body and how to prevent a low glucose level.

Exercise and Type 2 Diabetes

If you have type 2 diabetes, an exercise program can improve insulin sensitivity and lower your average blood glucose concentration. It also helps with weight loss and weight maintenance, provides cardiovascular benefits, and has the potential to lower blood pressure. Unlike individuals with type 1 diabetes, glucose regulation works in people with type 2, although some individuals with type 2 who take insulin or a medication that increases insulin secretion from the pancreas may have an occasional problem with low blood sugar.

Once you have gotten permission from your physician to exercise and there is nothing else that prevents you from exercising, your exercise program is then a matter of personal preference. It is important to do an exercise that you like to do and can easily access. You should think of exercise as an important component of your diabetes treatment, and it should be prescribed along with appropriate diet and medication.

Just like the pre-exercise checklist for type 1 diabetes, people with type 2 diabetes should also have a checklist that has been approved by their physician. Your physician may have more information that should be added to the checklist. See an example on the following page.

Example Pre-Exercise Checklist for People with Type 2

1. How long should I exercise and is this exercise appropriate?

   You should discuss the length and frequency of exercise with your physician.

2. Check to make sure you have your self-monitoring blood glucose test kit with plenty of test strips.

3. Do I need to test before exercise?

   If so, what glucose levels has your physician approved before, during, and after exercise?

4. Check to see that you have a snack and water if needed.

It is well known that exercise provides many benefits for individuals with diabetes. However, the goals and precautions for exercise are patient-specific, and may change over time depending on your blood glucose control. The American Diabetes Association (ADA) Standards of Medical Care in Diabetes recommends that "people with diabetes should be advised to perform at least 150 minutes/week of moderate-intensity aerobic physical activity (50 – 70% of maximum heart rate)." The ADA also recommends that, as long as there are no other conditions that make exercise inadvisable, people with type 2 should be encouraged to perform resistance training three times per week.

Exercise can be a very important component of your diabetes treatment, so I encourage you to start enjoying a physical activity soon, with the approval of your doctor. Try to make it something fun, and see if friends or family will join you so that your experience is even more enjoyable.

Summary

It is my firm belief that education about the disease is the first line of defense in understanding the reasons why these complications may develop and how to prevent them.

Just knowing that diabetes will progress to serious complications should be a strong enough incentive to learn as much as you can about the disease. Impaired fasting glucose and impaired glucose tolerance are pre-diabetic conditions that can progress to diabetes. Insulin is the body's "great communicator" and plays a part in directing the functions of many different body systems. Having diabetes and being overweight increases the likelihood of insulin resistance and can reduce insulin's ability to correctly send its signals throughout your body. Losing weight will help to increase your body's sensitivity to insulin.

The first steps to taking control of your diabetes include contacting your physician to go over your treatment plan and making sure all your tests are up to date. If you are overweight, begin tracking your calories and target an exercise program that will help you reach your goal weight.

I truly believe that you can take control of your diabetes when you have knowledge to do so. Diabetes should not stop you from doing the things you love in life, or from attaining your goals.

Facts at a Glance

1. **Diabetes** is a condition in which there is a buildup of sugar (glucose) in your bloodstream. The sugar comes from two sources: The breakdown of the food we eat and glucose produced by the liver. Uncontrolled diabetes will definitely lead to complications, such as heart problems, kidney problems, worsening or loss of sight, and amputations.

2. **Insulin** is a hormone that allows glucose into a cell so that it can be used for energy. Insulin is produced by the pancreas. It is like a key that unlocks the door of the cell and allows the glucose to go inside. Glucose can only provide energy to the body when it goes into a cell. If it cannot enter the cell, it will build up in the bloodstream and cells will be starved for energy.

3. **Insulin resistance** is a condition in which insulin does not work well. It is associated with being overweight. The more overweight you are, the more insulin resistant you become. Losing weight can help decrease insulin resistance.

Your Action Steps

This action plan is called ACT.

A > **Appointment:** Make an appointment with your physician or care provider. Go over your treatment plan with your physician.

Get a baseline or current measurement of your weight, blood pressure, a blood glucose test called A1C, cholesterol levels, and get permission to exercise. These baseline measurements will help you track your progress.

C > **Calories:** Eat three healthy, balanced meals a day.

Keep track of your calorie intake by learning how to read a nutrition label. Do not skip meals, as this has been shown to cause overeating. Eat two healthy snacks of less than 150 calories between meals to help curb your appetite. Chapter Six (page 157), Healthy Eating for People with Diabetes, has information on how to read nutrition labels, along with other healthy eating tips.

T > **Target:** Target an exercise program that will work for you.

Make sure to get your doctor's approval to start an exercise program and then try a few different activities to see what you like. Walking is easy and requires no special equipment. Whatever you choose, make sure it is something you enjoy and can easily access.

Chapter 2

What Is the Next Step?

Now that you understand what diabetes is and how to diagnose it, the next step is to learn about what you can do to keep your diabetes under control. We will discuss the ABCs of diabetes, why they are important and how to control them. This information builds the framework for the following chapters, which will go into the pathology (medical reasons) of why complications occur. By the time we discuss medications in Chapter 5, you will have a full cycle of knowledge about:

- What diabetes is
- Why complications arise
- Why it is important to have certain medical tests done
- How to prevent complications
- The reasons behind the choices of prescription medications

I know that at first it will be challenging to stay on top of your medications, get your lab tests done on time, and keep track of all the other things that are important to controlling diabetes, like diet and exercise. There is no doubt that it requires effort, perseverance, and commitment. At the same time, it is almost an understatement to say that life keeps all of us very busy. I know it seems like a lot. But I want to assure you that what may seem overwhelming now will not stay that way. It is only a matter of perception. What feels like an overwhelming number of tasks today will soon become second nature to you.

Think back to your first day of school. When you walked in the door that day, you probably were a bit worried: Where do I sit? What am I supposed to do? Who are all these kids? Will I be able to follow the rules? What ARE the rules!? But almost certainly within a few days or weeks, it was a piece of cake. You knew where to go and when to go there, you understood the classroom rules, what the teacher expected of you and how to do it! It was not hard anymore and maybe you even got a sense of satisfaction from figuring it all out. It is the same thing with learning to control your diabetes. It just takes some time to learn what you need to know and get comfortable with giving it a place in your life.

There is no time like the present, as the saying goes. It is tempting to think that you can wait until next week or next month to get that test you need or make an appointment with your doctor. As long as you feel fine there is no rush, right? Well, I can certainly say that it is true that there *is* always another day, but what will that day bring if you do not control your diabetes? The question really is what quality of life do you want to be experiencing tomorrow, next year, or ten years from now? Do you want to feel healthy and full of life, or ill and run down, possibly struggling with complications like kidney failure or vision loss? There really is no time like the present to make the commitment to yourself to having the healthiest future you can.

It is important that you take the initiative to learn about diabetes so that you can understand what your physician is saying and be able to ask good questions to clarify the information you are given. While I am certain that physicians want to do their best for every patient they see, it is simply not feasible for your doctor to spend an hour or two with you to educate you about diabetes. Doctors today are plagued by time constraints and a very high volume of patients, which makes it impossible for them to chase you down to make sure you get your tests done or that you are taking your medications. Can you imagine a physician trying to remember everyone he or she saw last month? Who needs to get a lab test? What prescriptions were ordered? Physicians document all this information in your chart, but they are simply unable to sit down and do a leisurely review of your records just to see if you are keeping up with your diabetes control. It is this reality that makes it so very important that you take charge of your medical care.

It is not hard to be proactive with your diabetes when you know the facts. I did an interview with my friend Paul who has type 1 diabetes to accommodate my first edition of a diabetes book I wrote. Paul related how he never truly educated himself about diabetes, was not given the information he needed by his physicians, and lived most of his life with his diabetes out of control. By the time Paul did take control of his diabetes and lost over 120 pounds, he had already passed 40 years of his life with uncontrolled glucose. Paul is now in kidney failure and gets dialysis treatments three times a week. He recently said to me, "If only someone told me what could happen." Now, in light of his very serious diabetic complications, Paul's wife says, "We have to learn how to live today so that we can live tomorrow."

I do not want what happened to Paul to happen to you. Take the time now to learn all you can about your diabetes, so that you can have many, many healthy tomorrows.

In-Depth Information

In chapter 1 you learned some of the fundamentals of diabetes. Chapters 3 and 4 will go into depth on the complications of diabetes and how to prevent them. In Chapters 5 and 6 you will learn about what questions to ask your physician and how to eat healthy to help control your diabetes. This chapter on the ABCs of Diabetes is meant to ease you into the educational component of controlling your diabetes, and familiarize you with some of the fundamentals of managing your disease. This information will make it easier to follow the upcoming chapters which provide more detail about why complications happen and how to control them.

Without education about your disease, you are ill-prepared to make informed decisions about your diabetes care or change your behavior. Ultimately, you may be poorly equipped to manage your diabetes effectively. Poor diabetes management will likely result in less than optimal health and the increased likelihood of developing complications. But education is only useful when it is turned into action; actually doing what you know you need to do to bring your diabetes under good control. The more you understand diabetes, the more important test results become, because they give you measurable points on what you have accomplished and what you need to change. This information gives you the power to be proactive and shows you where to concentrate your efforts. Tests are what you need to do in order to put your education into action.

To support this, I have developed an easy tool to help you remember the most important health points and their corresponding tests so that you can control your disease. It is called the ABCs of Diabetes.

The ABCs of Diabetes

A – A1C

B – Blood Pressure

C – Cholesterol

S – Smoking

The ABCs of Diabetes

A is for A1C. Your A1C is a measurement of the average amount of glucose that has been in your bloodstream over a three-month period. The lower your A1C value, the less glucose has been in your bloodstream over a three-month period, indicating how effective your glucose control was during that time. It is a blood test that is performed by a lab and is different than your home glucose monitoring. An A1C test gives you and your doctor an overview of how well you have controlled your blood glucose and shows whether or not you are on target or at goal.

For people with diabetes, The American Diabetes Association (ADA) recommends an A1C goal of less than 7%. Although many people with diabetes can follow the

ADA's recommendation, there are certain groups of people, such as children, pregnant women and the elderly who may require special consideration. If you are in one of these categories, your physician may determine a different goal for you. Having your A1C test done a minimum of twice a year provides important information for you and your physician. It is a tool that will help you and your doctor know how well your medication is working to achieve your goal, and whether or not you need to add another medication or increase the dose of existing medication to get to goal. Because high blood glucose causes many often severe complications, it is imperative to get your blood glucose under control, even if it takes two or three medications to accomplish that. **Note**: A1C testing should be done twice a year unless your glucose is not under control. In that case, it should be done every three months until your A1C is under control.

Your A1C test is a blood test done by a lab, but it directly correlates to your daily home blood glucose testing. The higher your blood glucose levels are at home, the higher your test results will be when you have your A1C evaluation at the lab. Figure 2.1 shows the relationship between A1C and blood glucose levels.

A1C Result	Blood Glucose
12	298
11	269
10	240
9	212
8	183
7	154
6	126

An A1C of 9 corresponds to an average glucose level of 212. Whether you have type 1 or type 2 diabetes, a blood glucose level of 212 is high; so is an A1C of 9. Also, because the A1C test is an average of your blood glucose levels over a three-month period of time, this means that at some point you may have had a glucose reading higher than 212, possibly 249, but you may also have had some low readings that counteracted the high reading resulting in an average of 212. There are multiple number combinations that can make up an average glucose that correspond to your A1C. See the following chart.

Table 6.1—Estimated average glucose (eAG)		
A1C (%)	mg/dL*	mmol/L
5	97 (76–120)	5.4 (4.2–6.7)
6	126 (100–152)	7.0 (5.5–8.5)
7	154 (123–185)	8.6 (6.8–10.3)
8	183 (147–217)	10.2 (8.1–12.1)
9	212 (170–249)	11.8 (9.4–13.9)
10	240 (193–282)	13.4 (10.7–15.7)
11	269 (217–314)	14.9 (12.0–17.5)
12	298 (240–347)	16.5 (13.3–19.3)

Data in parentheses are 95% CI. A calculator for converting A1C results into eAG, in either mg/dL or mmol/L, is available at professional.diabetes.org/eAG. *These estimates are based on ADAG data of 2,700 glucose measurements over 3 months per A1C measurement in 507 adults with type 1, type 2, or no diabetes. The correlation between A1C and average glucose was 0.92 (13,14). Adapted from Nathan et al. (13). ADA 2024

Diabetes Standard of Care 2023

In type 1 diabetes, the onset of symptoms can be so sudden and severe that many people are hospitalized when the disease first strikes. In contrast, when a person starts to develop type 2 diabetes, there are no strong symptoms that would alert you to see your doctor. Because of this, the diagnosis of type 2 is often delayed. By the time it is diagnosed, the disease has already progressed. As a result, about 50 percent of newly diagnosed type 2 patients already have evidence of early complications. Knowing that you may have had diabetes for years before your actual diagnosis should make you more proactive in frequent testing to ensure your blood glucose is in control. You are making up for lost time!

The important message here is that controlling your blood glucose is your highest priority in order to achieve good health. Over time, uncontrolled glucose will lead to complications, such as kidney, eye, and nerve disease. Conversely, lowering and controlling your blood glucose helps prevent or decrease the progression of these complications. Two large studies, the Diabetes Control and Complications Trial (DCCT) and the United Kingdom Prospective Diabetes Study (UKPDS) trials showed that better blood glucose control resulted in decreased complications. Understanding how important an A1C test is and how it provides your physician with good, measurable information on how to treat your diabetes should be a compelling reason to get this test done.

Do not let a high A1C result throw you off track. Instead, use your energy to work with your physician to figure out what you need to do to have better control of your diabetes. There is an old saying: "You can get bitter or better." I prefer the latter, get better.

The ABCs of Diabetes – Blood Pressure

B is for blood pressure. High blood pressure is called **hypertension**. Hypertension is a common condition of diabetes. As many as two out of three adults with diabetes also have hypertension. Hypertension is a major contributor (risk factor) for developing cardiovascular disease, kidney and eye disease, stroke, and nerve problems. Hypertension is often called "the silent killer" because you cannot feel it if you have it. There are often no symptoms you can detect on your own.

The American Diabetes Association (ADA) recommends blood pressure testing at every office visit with your doctor. Regular blood pressure checks at your physician's office, at home with your own blood pressure monitor, or other places that offer this service are essential in finding out if you have this condition so you can start treatment. Keep in mind that diagnosis of high blood pressure cannot be made with one measurement. It must be confirmed with repeat testing on separate days. Chapter 3 provides more details about how hypertension occurs, how it is diagnosed, and how this disease affects other body functions.

For individuals with diabetes, your goal blood pressure is **less than 130/80 mmHg** (millimeters of mercury), unless you have diabetes <u>and</u> kidney disease, in which case your physician may require a goal blood pressure of less than 125/70 mmHg.

Because hypertension affects so many organs and body systems, getting your blood pressure to goal is a key element to preventing complications. While changing your habits such as diet and exercise may help you lower your blood pressure, most individuals with diabetes will require medication; sometimes two or three if your blood pressure is ≥ 160/100 mmHg to achieve their goal. There are many blood pressure medications that combine two drugs into one tablet to make this easier. Make it a point to check with your doctor to see whether or not you have achieved your goal.

The ABCs of Diabetes – Cholesterol

C is for cholesterol. Cholesterol is a soft, waxy substance found in your bloodstream and in all your body's cells. Cholesterol cannot be dissolved in the blood and a buildup of cholesterol can lead to atherosclerosis. Atherosclerosis comes from the Greek words *athero*, meaning paste, and *sclerosis*, meaning hardness. Therefore, your arteries can get a buildup of cholesterol that can cause plaque and can lead to heart problems, such as heart attacks and stroke. As cholesterol builds up on the walls of your arteries, it becomes more difficult for your blood to flow through them. The danger of cholesterol build up is twofold:

- first, it causes a decrease in your blood flow

- second, a piece of cholesterol may break off and travel through your arteries until it gets stuck in a small blood vessel and blocks blood flow, causing a heart attack or stroke.

The ADA recommends that your cholesterol levels be checked at least once a year. This is done with a blood test performed at a lab that will provide four results: total cholesterol, LDL (Low Density Lipoproteins), HDL

(High Density Lipoproteins), and triglycerides. These four components are part of the body's system that influence cholesterol metabolism and establishes the presence or absence of possible disease-producing capability. Here is a description of each of these components and the goals for people with diabetes as developed by the ADA, which updates them yearly. Your physician may set different goals for you depending on your health. Table 2.2 on page 59 sets out the desired goals for each component of your cholesterol results.

Total Cholesterol

Total cholesterol is a value that is a composite of all the components of your cholesterol screening: LDL, HDL, and triglycerides.

Total Cholesterol Goal: Below 200 mg/dl

HDL and LDL

Because cholesterol cannot be dissolved in your body, it has to be carried to and from your cells by two lipoproteins, HDL and LDL. High density lipoprotein (HDL) carries cholesterol away from the bloodstream to the liver to help prevent cholesterol build up in arteries, and is referred to as the "good cholesterol." An easy way to remember that HDL is the good cholesterol carrier is that H stands for high grades, and we all want high grades. Your goal is to achieve a high value for HDL.

HDL Goals: Men = greater than 40 mg/dl Women = greater than 50 mg/dl

Low density lipoprotein (LDL) is made from very low

density lipoprotein (VLDL) that carries cholesterol from your liver into your bloodstream where it is deposited into your arteries. LDL is referred to as the "bad cholesterol." A good way to remember this is that L stands for low grades. Your goal is low LDL value.

LDL Goals: Less than 100 mg/dl; if you have heart disease, then 70 mg/dl

Triglycerides

Triglycerides are the form in which most fat exists in food and in your body. Any calories you eat that are not used for energy are converted to triglycerides to be stored as fat in your body. Excess triglycerides are linked to heart disease in some people.

Triglyceride Goal: Less than 150 mg/dl.

Cholesterol Goals Table	
Total Cholesterol	Less than 200 mg/dl
HDL (good cholesterol)	Greater than: Males: 40 mg/dl Females: 50 mg/dl
LDL (bad cholesterol)	Less than: Diabetes only: 100 mg/dl Diabetes and heart disease: 70 mg/dl
Triglycerides	Less than: 150 mg/dl

Table 2.2

People with diabetes are two to four times more likely to develop heart disease, so it is important to control your cholesterol. The only way to know if you are in control is to get a cholesterol test.

Once you know your numbers, you can determine if you need to make any changes to bring your results within goal. There are many different ways you can work on improving cholesterol results such as:

- diet
- reducing saturated fats and cholesterol in the foods you eat
- increasing your daily fiber intake by eating more fruits and vegetables
- and exercise
- 30 minutes a day most days of the week

Medication may also be an option to help you get within range.

Many studies have shown that a group of medications called statins are excellent at decreasing LDL, which the ADA says is the primary cholesterol lowering goal for people with diabetes. Cholesterol control and medications are discussed in greater detail in the next chapter, including a list of medications. You can bring the list with you to your doctor's office so that you can review which medication is right for you.

The ABCS of Diabetes – Smoking

S is for smoking. The ADA suggests that any person with diabetes should try to stop smoking. Smoking causes many adverse affects in the body that are probably not felt, but may also contribute to worsening of complications that already exist. People who smoke a pack of cigarettes a day have more than twice the risk of heart attack than non-smokers.

Nicotine from cigarettes causes your blood vessels to constrict, or squeeze, and elevates your blood pressure by five to ten points. This may make it that much more difficult to get to goal with your blood pressure, putting you at risk for complications. A study at Johns Hopkins Medical Institutions showed smoking can cause hypertension and weakening of the left ventricle of the heart in people who previously had no symptoms of high blood pressure. Smoking can affect the heart by increasing your heart rate, decreasing oxygen delivery, and putting more stress on your heart from high blood pressure. Blood clot formation is also increased, which in turn increases the potential for heart attack and stroke. Women who smoke and also take birth control pills increase their risk of heart attack, stroke and peripheral vascular disease which is the name for obstruction of arteries in the kidneys, stomach, arms, legs or feet. Your heart, eyes, kidneys, and nerves are all affected by high blood pressure, increasing the potential of developing complications.

With this knowledge, you can see how dangerous it is to smoke if you have diabetes. Since individuals with diabetes are already two to four times more likely to develop heart disease, smoking is like touching a stove that is on to see if it is hot.

Smoking cessation, or quitting, is not easy, but there are products that can help you quit. Make sure to discuss these products with your physician. All Food and Drug Administration (FDA) approved drugs for smoking cessation show more than twice the quit rate of success over trying to quit on your own. FDA products that contain nicotine have also been shown to be superior in helping people to stop smoking. Some of these aids require a prescription and others are available over-the-counter. Discussing your options with your doctor about what is best for you is a good idea.

Summary

High blood glucose, high blood pressure, and cholesterol are the main contributors to the development of complications in people with diabetes. You just need to make the decision that you are ready to do what it takes to control your diabetes in order to eliminate any possibility of complications.

When diabetes is not controlled unfortunately, the natural progression of uncontrolled diabetes is to cause complications that will eventually lead to illness or death. That is why it is so important to understand complications and know how to prevent or slow their progression so that they do not interfere with your life and health.

This process is called Optimal Life because you can lead an optimal life even if you have diabetes and if you know how to keep yourself healthy. There are no magic pills, but with greater understanding of diabetes and why you should follow the steps outlined in this book, there is no reason your diabetes should prevent you from living your life to the fullest.

Facts at a Glance

The ABCS

A> **A1C:** A1C is a blood glucose test to measure the average glucose (sugar) that has been in your bloodstream over a three-month period of time. This test is done at the lab and is different than your glucose testing at home. It should be performed at least twice a year if your diabetes is controlled. If your diabetes is not controlled, an A1C should be done 4 times a year. The American Diabetes Association (ADA) recommends an A1C goal of less than 7%.

B> **Blood Pressure:** Blood pressure is a measurement of blood's pressure on your arteries when your heart contracts and relaxes. Your blood pressure should be less than 130/80 mmHg and you should have it measured every time you go to your doctor's office. Keeping your blood pressure under control decreases the risk of heart and kidney disease.

C> **Cholesterol:** Cholesterol is a soft waxy substance found in lipids (fats) in the bloodstream and is found in all your body's cells. When your cholesterol is measured at the lab, it will have four components: total cholesterol, LDL, HDL, and triglycerides. Your cholesterol levels should fall within the following ranges according to the ADA:

- **Total cholesterol** should be less than 200 mg/dl.

- **LDL** = This is the bad cholesterol (L--think of low grades) and should be less than 100 mg/dl. If you have heart problems, a lower goal of less than 70 mg/dl may be recommended if you have existing heart problems.

- **HDL** = This is the good cholesterol (H--think of high grades) and should be greater than 40 mg/dl for men, and greater than 50 mg/dl for women.

- **Triglycerides** are a type of fat found in your blood. Your triglyceride count should be less than 150 mg/dl.

S> **Smoking:** Smoking is harmful to everyone but is particularly bad for people with diabetes. It constricts your blood vessels, increasing your heart rate and blood pressure, and contributes to the formation of blood clots. If you smoke, create a plan to quit as soon as possible.

Your Three Action Steps

1. Check your blood sugar (glucose) level.

   - Get a glucose monitor (glucometer) and learn how to use it properly. Check your blood sugar on a daily basis. Your physician will tell you when and how often to check each day.

   - Get an A1C test twice a year. You can ask your physician to order this test for you. If you are not at goal, you should have this test performed every three months.

2. Check your blood pressure frequently.

   - You can do this at your physician's office, your local pharmacy, purchase it independently, or see if your health insurance will provide you with a blood pressure monitor to use at home.

- If your blood pressure is greater than 130/80 mmHg, ask your doctor if you need medication.

3. Get your cholesterol checked once a year.

- You can ask your physician to order a cholesterol panel for you.

- Check to see if you are at goal for total cholesterol, LDL, HDL, and triglycerides. If you are not, ask if you need to be on medication.

Chapter 3

How Do I Prevent Complications of Blood Pressure, Cholesterol, and Low Blood Sugar?

Introduction

You have now gained a foundation in the complex body systems affected by diabetes. I hope you see that taking an active role in your own health is by far the most important thing you can do. In this chapter, we will go into greater depth on the pathology and consequences of high blood pressure, heart problems, cholesterol, and low blood sugar. I think that having this information is not only interesting for its own sake, but it will also help you in your quest to prevent complications and give you understanding as to why certain medications are prescribed.

I believe this point in the series is where you start to become an expert on your disease and really gain insight into why you need to do the right thing and take care of yourself.

For cholesterol, we start right at the beginning with:

- what happens when you eat a meal
- following it through your body's systems to where it may begin to cause problems.

On blood pressure, we begin with:

- the pressure blood applies to the blood vessels
- how blood pressure affects different organs and discuss the body's truly amazing system for controlling blood pressure.

Low blood glucose is also discussed. You will learn:

- how it can happen
- how to prevent it
- and what to do when your blood glucose is low.

I am excited that you have made it this far in the book, because I know that this knowledge will help you change the way you make decisions about controlling your diabetes.

Knowledge is power and once you learn something, it is hard to go back to your old ways. I recently had a conversation with an individual managing type 2 diabetes while caring for a young child. Upon receiving his diagnosis, he felt understandably concerned about potential complications. In response, he took a proactive step by reorganizing his refrigerator and cupboards, opting for healthier food choices. This simple but powerful decision led to a remarkable transformation that marked the beginning of his wellness journey. Today, he is 100 pounds lighter, full of energy, and enjoying a vibrant life. His story shows how mindful choices can lead to extraordinary results.

Consider this story as an inspiring example of how small changes can lead to significant improvements in health and vitality. As we explore more about heart health and cholesterol in the next section, you may discover your own path to making beneficial changes that work for you and your lifestyle.

Blood Pressure

Controlling your blood pressure and keeping it within a healthy range is especially important for people with diabetes. Not only does high blood pressure (hypertension) pose a significant health risk in and of itself, but it can also accelerate other complications of diabetes, such as kidney and heart disease. Approximately 80 percent of people with type 2 diabetes also have hypertension.

Heart disease is a common cause of death in individuals with hypertension, and since diabetes already increases the risk of heart disease two times to four times more, you can see that controlling hypertension is a must. The risk of heart disease increases with each elevation in your blood pressure. Because hypertension often has no symptoms until serious complications have already occurred, it is often called the "silent killer." This makes it especially important that you know your numbers and check your blood pressure frequently.

What Is High Blood Pressure?

When your blood pressure is above normal, it is called hypertension. High blood pressure (hypertension) occurs when:

1. your blood vessels are narrowed or constricted,

2. there is an increase in fluid retained in the body making your heart work harder, or

3. a combination of the two.

Blood pressure is a measurement of how much force blood puts on the walls of your blood vessels. When you have your blood pressure measured, the reading will be given in two numbers:

- The Systolic (SBP) measurement. The systolic (top number) reading measures pressure when your heart contracts to pump the blood.

- The Diastolic (DBP) measurement. The diastolic (bottom number) reading measures pressure when your heart is at rest between beats.

A normal blood pressure reading is less than 120/80 mmHg (milligrams of mercury). Verbally, this would be expressed as 120 over 80.

Both the American Diabetes Association (ADA) and the American Heart Association (AHA) have defined the ranges for healthy blood pressure, depending on whether or not you have diabetes. Take a look at Table 3.1, which shows the different stages of high blood pressure. For people who do not have diabetes, the American College of Cardiology guidelines changed the definition of hypertension of blood pressure from greater than 140/90 to greater than 130/80 mmHg in the U.S.A., but in Europe it is still defined as greater than 140/90 mmHg. However, people with diabetes have an even stricter standard, which is less than 130/80 mmHg. If you have diabetes and kidney disease, your goal blood pressure may be as low as 125/75 mmHg.

Normal Blood Pressure	<120	<80
Elevated Blood Pressure	120-129	<80
Stage 1 hypertension	130-139	80-89
Stage 2 hypertension	≥140	≥90
Isolated systolic hypertension	≥140	<90
Diabetes goal	<130	<80
Diabetes + Low ASCVD Risk	<130	<80
Diabetes + Higher ASCVD Risk	<140	<90

Table 3.1 Different stages of high blood pressure.
American Diabetes Association: Standards of Medical Care in Diabetes—2022.
ACC/AHA recommend a Universal Blood Pressure Goal of <130/80 mmHg
Higher ASCVD Risk: Higher cardiovascular risk, means those with existing ASCVD (Atherosclerotic Cardiovascular Disease) or 10-year ASCVD risk ≥15%.

How High Blood Pressure Affects Diabetes

High blood pressure affects every organ in your body and the relationship between insulin resistance and hypertension is well established. One of insulin's many effects in the body is:

- that it opens blood vessels by relaxing their muscular walls called vasodilatory,

- with secondary effects on sodium or salt reabsorption in the kidneys.

When you have insulin resistance:

- the vasodilation effect of insulin is lost,

- but the reabsorption of sodium by the kidneys is still functioning.

This means your blood vessels are not widening but salt uptake is still occurring. With increased sodium absorption, there is an increased risk of water retention in the bloodstream. Extra water puts pressure on your circulatory system and increases blood pressure.

As high blood pressure progresses, it puts stress on your heart by making it work harder to push blood into narrow or constricted arteries. Over time, your heart muscle weakens because the continual stress causes the heart muscle to enlarge with fibrous tissue, making it weak and stiff. This is called remodeling because the heart changes shape as it gets larger. If high blood pressure continues uncontrolled, heart failure will set in due to the inability of the heart to pump adequate blood supplies into the bloodstream. Hypertension is also a risk factor for brain stroke and bleeding. The incidence of stroke rises as blood pressure increases, especially in individuals over the age of 65.

Hypertension also adversely affects your kidneys. Studies have shown that people who have blood pressure greater than 130/80 mmHg have a greater likelihood of developing end-stage kidney disease. Your kidneys are highly vascular meaning there are many blood vessels. The blood vessels act as tiny filtering units that take materials and excess water out of the bloodstream that need to be urinated out and retain the elements that should stay in your body. Uncontrolled high blood pressure on these tiny filtering vessels of the kidney eventually causes injury or destruction. When this happens, your kidneys cannot filter fluid as well as before and fluid begins to accumulate in your system, which in turn increases high blood pressure.

Your eyes are also sensitive to blood pressure, as they also are comprised of many tiny blood vessels. Extra stress on the blood vessels of your eyes can cause your retinae to dilate and detach; the small vessels may burst and bleed, causing your eyesight to deteriorate. This type of eye disease is known as hypertensive retinopathy and the damage can be serious.

High Blood Pressure and Being Overweight

The more overweight you are, the more fat (adipose) tissue you have, resulting in more free fatty acids (FFAs) being released into your bloodstream. Free fatty acids reduce the ability of your muscles to take up glucose for energy. Your muscles start to become insulin resistant by:

- slowing down the ability of insulin-mediated glucose uptake into the cells

- resulting in increased blood glucose levels.

The buildup of glucose in the circulation increases the demand for insulin secretion on the pancreas and results in excess insulin in the blood called hyperinsulinemia.

Hyperinsulinemia leads to:

- increased sodium retention

- and increased adrenalin and noradrenalin production from your nervous system

- which contributes to hypertension.

Additionally, this effect causes the blood vessels to narrow and constrict, thus putting more pressure on blood vessels and the heart. Here again you can see the relationship between fluid retention, blood vessel constriction, and blood pressure.

Hormonal system called The Renin-Angiotensin-Aldosterone System Effect on High Blood Pressure (RAAS System)

The renin-angiotensin-aldosterone system, which is also called the RAAS system, is made up of a complex balance of hormones that work together to regulate your blood pressure. Your kidneys primarily regulate this system. The RAAS system regulates sodium, potassium, and fluid balance that impact the amount of water retained which increases the blood volume and contributes to high blood pressure in your body. The fluid or blood volume affects how hard your heart needs to pump as well as constriction of the arteries which increases high blood pressure.

Blood volume is controlled by a delicate balance of the amount of water and salt that contains sodium taken in through food and drink and the amount of liquid excreted by the kidneys into the urine. To maintain blood volume within a normal range, the kidneys regulate the amount of water and sodium passed into the urine. For example, if excessive water and salt (sodium) are ingested, the kidneys normally respond by excreting more water and sodium into the urine. This is necessary because too much blood volume increases blood pressure, putting extra strain on the heart.

The opposite happens if your kidneys sense that your blood fluid volume is low, they activate the RAAS system. This triggers a series of events, including the release of another hormone, aldosterone, which causes an increase of the amount of sodium to be retained and a decrease in the amount of water to be passed into urine. An easy way to remember this process is that water follows sodium. If sodium is retained in the body by the kidneys, water will also stay in the body. You may notice an increase in water retention after a really salty meal. Your hands may swell and your rings may feel tight, or your feet may swell and your shoes may feel too small.

Through the RAAS system and its complex, delicate interactions, your body constantly monitors and adjusts the volume, and thus the pressure of the fluids flowing through your body. When the RAAS is working optimally, healthy blood pressure levels are maintained.

How to Prevent and Control High Blood Pressure

Lose Weight – Losing 22 pounds (10kg) can reduce your blood pressure 5 to 20 points. This is because the more overweight or obese you are, the more strain is placed on your heart and arteries by increasing fluid volume, causing your kidneys to work harder, which can lead to albumin (protein) loss and progressive kidney dysfunction. As we have already learned, the increase in fluid increases the pressure on your kidneys, makes your heart work harder, and can cause constriction of your blood vessels. This, in turn, can activate hormones that lead to high blood pressure.

Exercise - Increased physical activity helps your circulation, strengthens your heart, and aids in weight loss.

Healthy Eating - The DASH diet (Dietary Approaches to Stop Hypertension) was developed by the National

Institutes of Health as an eating plan for people with hypertension. It is rich in fruits, vegetables, and low-fat dairy products, with a reduced content of saturated and total fat. Incorporating the eating habits described in the DASH diet can further decrease blood pressure by 8 to 14 mmHg. Additionally, decreasing the amount of salt in your food, both the salt you put on and the salt used in commercial processing, will help reduce water weight gain. It is important to keep water weight gain in check because excess water in your circulatory system causes an increase in the volume of fluid your heart has to pump, which puts extra stress on it. Chapter 7, Healthy Eating for People with Diabetes, shows you how to read a food label and gives you other tips for a good diet.

Another way to lower your blood pressure is to avoid caffeine or decrease the amount you drink. Caffeine can cause a short but dramatic increase in blood pressure, even if you do not normally have high blood pressure. 200 mg of caffeine can raise systolic blood pressure 3 to 14 mmHg and diastolic blood pressure 4 to 13 mmHg. A cup of coffee has about 100 mg of caffeine. To see if caffeine might be raising your blood pressure, check your blood pressure within 30 minutes of drinking a cup of coffee or other caffeinated beverage you regularly consume. If your blood pressure increases by five to ten points, you may be sensitive to the blood pressure raising effects of caffeine. If you choose to reduce your intake of caffeine, do so gradually over several days to a week to avoid withdrawal headaches.

Monitoring how much alcohol you drink will also lower your blood pressure. Alcohol raises blood pressure by increasing adrenaline-type hormones in your blood plasma.

Smoking - Cigarette smoking raises blood pressure by increasing hormones like norepinephrine, a substance related to adrenaline. These hormones cause your blood vessels to constrict, resulting in elevated blood pressure.

Figure 3.2 was developed by the National Heart, Lung, and Blood Institute (NHLBI) and the Seventh Report of the Joint National Committee on Prevention, Detection, Evaluation, and Treatment of High Blood Pressure. It shows the ways that different lifestyle modifications can lower blood pressure.

(See next page.)

Lifestyle Modifications and Blood Pressure		
Modification	**Recommendation**	**Approximate Systolic BP Reduction Range**
Weight reduction	Maintain normal body weight (BMI 18.5-24.9)	5-20 mmHg per 10 kg weight loss
Adopt DASH eating plan	Consume a diet rich in fruits, vegetables, and low fat dairy products with a reduced content of saturated and total fat	8-14 mmHg
Dietary Sodium reduction	Reduce dietary sodium intake to no more than 100 mEq/L (2.4 grams sodium, 6 grams sodium chloride)	2-8 mmHg
Physical activity	Engage in regular aerobic physical activity such as brisk walking at least 30 minutes per day most days of the week	4-9 mmHg
Moderation of alcohol consumption	Limit consumption to no more than 2 drinks per day (1 oz or 30 mL ethanol e.g., 24 oz beer, 10 oz wine, or 3 oz 80 proof whiskey) in most men, and no more than 1 drink per day in women and lighter weight persons	2-4 mmHg

Figure 3.2 Lifestyle modifications and lower blood pressure

Abbreviations: BMI, body mass index calculated as weight in kilograms divided by the square of height in meters; BP, blood pressure; DASH, Dietary Approaches to Stop Hypertension.

*For overall cardiovascular risk reduction, stop smoking.

The effects of implementing these modifications are dose and time dependent and could be higher for some individuals.

How to Get the Most Accurate Blood Pressure Reading

Whether you measure your blood pressure at home or at your doctor's office, it is important that you pay attention to some basic requirements, so your blood pressure readings are accurate. First, make sure the cuff goes around at least 80 percent of your arm. Your readings should be taken after you have been resting comfortably, back supported in the sitting or lying position, for at least five minutes, and you have not been smoking or drinking coffee within approximately 30 minutes. While your blood pressure is being measured, do not eat, drink, or talk until the reading is complete.

Blood Pressure Medications

When lifestyle changes are not enough to get you to goal, talk to your physician about starting medications. Most major guidelines strongly suggest that individuals with diabetes and hypertension may need two or more drugs to achieve their goal, and that thiazide diuretics, ACE (angiotensin converting enzyme) inhibitors, and ARBs (angiotensin II receptor blockers) are the first line of drugs to try. ACE inhibitors and ARBs are the most common; each works in the RAAS to moderate blood pressure.

Figure 3.3 presents a list of some of the most common medications.

(See following pages)

Medications for Hypertension		
Angiotensin-Converting Enzyme Inhibitors (ACE-Is)	Lotensin	benazepril
	Capoten	captopril
	Vasotec	enalapril
	Monopril	fosinopril
	Prinivil, Zestril	lisinopril
	Univasc	moexipril
	Aceon	perindopril
	Accupril	quinapril
	Altace	ramipril
	Mavik	trandolapril
Angiotensin-Converting Enzyme Inhibitors (ACE-Is) Combinations (continued on next page)	Lotrel	amlodipine/benazepril
	Lotensin HCT	benazepril/HCTZ
	Capozide	captopril/HCTZ
	Lexxel	enalapril/felodipine
	Vaseretic	enalapril/HCTZ
	Monopril HCT	fosinopril/HCTZ
	Prinzide, Zestoretic	lisinopril/HCTZ
	Uniretic	moexipril/HCTZ
	Accuretic	quinapril/HCTZ

Medications for Hypertension		
Angiotensin II Receptor Blockers (ARBs)	Edarbi	azilsartan
	Atacand	candesartan
	Avapro	irbesartan
	Cozaar	losartan
	Benicar	olmesartan
	Micardis	telmisartan
	Diovan	valsartan
Angiotensin II Receptor Blockers (ARBs) **Combinations**	Valturna	aliskiren/valsartan
	Exforge	amlodipine/valsartan
	Teveten HCT	candesartan/HCTZ
	Hyzaar	losartan/HCTZ
	AZOR	olmesartan/ amlodipine
	Tribenzor	olmesartan/ amlodipine/HCTZ
	Micardis HCT	telmisartan/HCTZ
	Twynsta	telmisartan/ amlodipine
	Diovan HCT	valsartan/HCTZ

On the next page, Figure 3.4 presents a list of some of the most common medications. Not a comprehensive list.

Calcium Channel Blockers	Katerzia	amlodipine benzoate
	Norvasc	amlodipine besylate
	Cardizem CD, Cardizem LA, Cartia XT, Diltzac, Tiazac, and Taztia XT	diltiazem
	Generic Medicine Only	felodipine
	Generic Medicine Only	isradipine
	Conjupri	levamlodipine
	Adalat CC and Procardia X	nifedipine
	Sular	nisoldipine
	Calan SR, Verelan, and Verelan PM	verapamil
Renin Inhibitors	Aliskiren	Tekturna

Diuretics (Sometimes called "water pills)	Midamor	Amiloride and hydrochlorothiazide
	Diuril	chlorothiazide
	Generic Medicine Only	chlorthalidone
	Inspra	eplerenone
	Lasix	furosemide
	Microzide	hydrochlorothiazide
	Aldactazide	hydrochlorothiazide and spironolactone
	Dyazide, Maxzide and Maxzide 25	hydrochlorothiazide and triamterene
	Generic Medicine Only	indapamide
	Aldactone and CaroSpir	spironolactone
	Demadex	torsemide
	Zaroxolyn	metolazone

Figure 3.4 —Most common medications (continued)

	Generic Medicine Only	acebutolol
	Tenormin	atenolol
	Generic Medicine Only	betaxolol
	Generic Medicine Only	bisoprolol
Beta Blockers	Coreg	carvedilol
	Coreg CR	carvedilol phosphate
	Trandate	labetalol
	Kapspargo Sprinkle and Toprol-XL	metoprolol succinate
	Lopressor	metoprolol tartrate
	Corgard	nadolol
	Bystolic	nebivolol
	Generic Medicine Only	pindolol
	Inderal, Inderal LA, and InnoPran XL	propranolol
	Generic Medicine Only	timolol

Combination Medications	Tekturna HCT	Aliskiren and hydrochlorothiazide
	Exforge	amlodipine besylate and valsartan
	Lotrel	amlodipine besylate and benazepril
	Azor	amlodipine besylate and olmesartan
	Prestalia	amlodipine besylate and perindopril
	Twynsta	amlodipine besylate and telmisartan
	Exforge HCT	Amlodipine besylate, hydrochlorothiazide, and valsartan
	Tenoretic 50, Tenoretic 100	Atenolol and chlorthalidone

Figure 3.4 —Most common medications (continued)

Combination Medications	Lotensin HCT	Benazepril and hydrochlorothiazide
	Atacand HCT	Candesartan and hydrochlorothiazide
	Generic Medicine Only	Captopril and hydrochlorothiazide
	Vaseretic	Enalapril and hydrochlorothiazide
	Generic Medicine Only	Fosinopril and hydrochlorothiazide
	Avalide	hydrochlorothiazide and irbesartan
	Zestoretic	hydrochlorothiazide and lisinopril
	Dutoprol	hydrochlorothiazide and metoprolol succinate
	Lopressor HCT	hydrochlorothiazide and metoprolol tartrate
	Benicar HCT	hydrochlorothiazide and olmesartan

Figure 3.4 —Most common medications (continued)

Combination Medications	Lopressor HCT	hydrochlorothiazide and metoprolol tartrate
	Benicar HCT	hydrochlorothiazide and olmesartan
	Accuretic and Quinaretic	hydrochlorothiazide and quinapril
	Micardis HCT	hydrochlorothiazide and telmisartan
	Ziac	Bisoprolol and hydrochlorothiazide

Combination Medications	Hyzaar	hydrochlorothiazide and losartan
	Generic Medicine Only	hydrochlorothiazide and metoprolol tartrate
	Generic Medicine Only	hydrochlorothiazide and moexipril
	Tribenzor	Amlodipine besylate, hydrochlorothiazide, and olmesartan
	Tarka	Trandolapril and verapamil
	Diovan HCT	hydrochlorothiazide and valsartan
	Edarbyclor	Chlorthalidone and zilsartan

Cholesterol and Cardiovascular Disease

It is a well-documented fact that people with type 1 and type 2 diabetes have an increased risk of cardiovascular (heart) disease, with as much as a two to four times increase in coronary heart disease (CHD). The landmark Framingham Heart Study revealed a marked increase in heart related events, such as coronary artery disease (cholesterol and plaque in the arteries), heart attacks, coronary heart failure in individuals with diabetes mellitus. The American Heart Association (AHA) has designated diabetes mellitus as a major risk factor for cardiovascular disease. Overall, coronary heart disease is the leading cause of death in individuals with diabetes over the age of 35.

With the overwhelming evidence confirming the correlation between diabetes and the increased risk of heart disease, people with diabetes must pay close attention to this potential complication. So, what do you do? Cholesterol control is important to prevent the buildup of fatty plaque in your arteries that can lead to circulation and heart problems, a process leading to **atherosclerosis.**

Atherosclerosis is a condition where the fatty components of cholesterol form deposits along the walls of your arteries and can develop into fibrosis, plaque formation and calcification. As this condition develops, normal blood flow is decreased, leading to poor circulation. As the condition worsens, small pieces of cholesterol plaque can break off and flow through the bloodstream until they come to a blood vessel that is too small to allow the piece of plaque to continue. The plaque blocks the blood vessel so there is little or no blood flow. The decrease in blood flow also decreases the delivery of oxygen in the area of the blocked blood vessel. Decreased or no oxygen in a blood vessel is termed ischemia. This can happen in the heart (heart attack) or the brain (stroke) and cause cell death in these areas.

It's entirely possible that you may not feel these small artery blockages, and there may be no symptoms of chest pain. This is called silent ischemia and it is common in individuals with diabetes. The danger of silent ischemia is that you do not know when it may evolve and worsen, causing a heart attack or stroke. It's like a ticking time bomb waiting to explode.

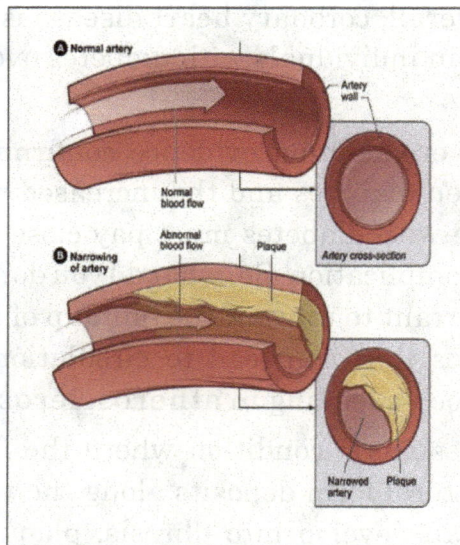

Figure 3.4 A depiction of atherosclerosis. Source: By NHLBI [Public domain], via Wikimedia Commons

How Does Cholesterol Build Up in Your Body?

There are several reasons why cholesterol build up may occur, such as diet, a genetic predisposition, or a combination of both. To see the whole picture, let us start with what happens when we eat. The fats that come from the food we eat are delivered to the bloodstream via the intestines and liver. So, after having a meal, the triglycerides (fat) and cholesterol that were in the food are absorbed by the small intestine. The triglycerides and cholesterol are packaged into small particles called chylomicrons, and find their way into the blood.

The more fatty foods you eat, the more free fatty acids are produced in the body that will eventually be taken up by your body. The more fat that is taken up by your tissues, the more overweight you become. As noted previously, being overweight is directly associated with insulin resistance. Some studies even suggest that chylomicron formation which is the fat and cholesterol in the intestine may also be increased in insulin resistant type 2 diabetes. Studies have also shown that an increased flow of FFAs to the liver can increase the production of bad cholesterol that will be released into the bloodstream and become LDL, the "bad cholesterol."

What are LDL and HDL

LDL and HDL are both lipoproteins, meaning they contain fat (lipo) and a protein, and are referred to as carrier lipoproteins. The bad cholesterol called VLDL-LDL carries fat into the blood from the liver. The good cholesterol called HDL carries the fat out of the blood circulation back to the liver. The connection between the fats we eat or make in the body is in the form of triglycerides, the chemical form in which most fat exists in food, as well as in the body. Therefore, ingesting food with high fat content increases blood triglycerides, placing a burden on the body to direct and get rid of the fat. The danger of having high LDL in the bloodstream is that it carries fats from the liver into the blood, which can be deposited in the arteries. The major structural protein component of LDL cholesterol is called **APOB** and is responsible for carrying cholesterol to the tissues. High levels of **APOB** can lead to atherosclerosis which is a disease of the arteries characterized by the deposits of plaque of fatty material on the arteries inner walls that causes vascular disease, leading to heart disease.

The danger of having low good cholesterol called HDL is that this lipoprotein carries cholesterol from the arteries and blood circulation back to the liver. The lower your HDL level, the more cholesterol is left in your bloodstream to be deposited in arteries. The higher the HDL the more cholesterol is taken out of the blood and back to the liver. The major structural protein component of HDL is APOA, which picks up cholesterol from the circulation or tissues and brings it back to the liver to be metabolized and removed from the blood system. That is why it is so important to take steps to elevate your HDL cholesterol levels. The higher your HDL level, the greater protection you have from atherosclerosis.

Insulin Resistance and Cholesterol

One of the roles of insulin in the liver is to target the LDL protein APOB to metabolize and eliminate it rather than release it into the bloodstream along with cholesterol. This is important because the APOB protein carries the bad cholesterol back out to the blood circulation. LDL triglyceride levels are commonly elevated in individuals with type 2 diabetes. Individuals with type 1 who have good blood glucose control usually have good triglyceride levels. It is believed this is because the insulin taken by type 1 individuals inhibits APOB secretion from the liver.

A major contributor to the body's insulin resistance is the fact that the less efficiently insulin works in the body, the greater the breakdown of fats that lead to free fatty acids. Increasing levels of free fatty acids in the body decreases the signaling mechanism that allows insulin to find the lock on the cell so it can open the door that allows glucose to enter. This insulin resistance decreases the ability of insulin to stop the liver from producing glucose. Additionally, FFAs increase the accumulation of triglycerides in both skeletal and cardiac muscle.

This becomes a vicious cycle where high blood glucose causes glucose to stick to lipoproteins, modifying them so they interact less efficiently in the body. Consequently, more cholesterol will stay in the bloodstream. At the same time, eating high fat foods releases FFAs into the bloodstream, where it is either taken up by adipose (fat) tissue or by muscle tissue. Adipose tissue takes the FFAs and makes triglyceride.

How to Prevent and Control High Cholesterol

So, again, the question is what can you do? As with your diabetes and glucose levels, the key to prevention of high cholesterol and its complications is to know your numbers. You should have a blood test performed by a laboratory yearly. Your doctor will need to order this test for you. It will show the total amount of cholesterol and will also give you values for high density lipoprotein (HDL), low density lipoprotein (LDL) and triglycerides.

Following are the guidelines for your ideal cholesterol levels as determined by the ADA:

Total cholesterol at or below 200 mg/dl

HDL above 40 mg/dl for males; at or below 50 mg/dl for females

LDL less than 100 mg/dl unless you already have heart disease; then it is suggested that your goal should be less than 70 mg/dl

Triglycerides less than 150 mg/dl

People with diabetes commonly have normal to high LDL, low HDL, and high triglycerides. Thus, the goal of your cholesterol control is to reverse this picture so that your bad cholesterol LDL is low. This is the lipoprotein that transports fats into your bloodstream; you want less of this. Your good cholesterol HDL is high. This is the lipoprotein that carries cholesterol away from your bloodstream; you want more of this. Your triglycerides are low. Triglycerides are the chemical form in which most fats exist in food, as well as in the body.

Once you know your numbers, you can make a plan for what you need to do in terms of diet, exercise, and medication so you can take control and decrease your risk of heart problems. An important first step in determining your action plan is to sit down with your physician when you get your lab results and review these numbers. If any of your numbers are higher than goal, you will want to develop a plan to bring them into a healthy range. One of the fastest ways to get control is through medication, but diet, exercise, quitting smoking, and other lifestyle changes can also substantially help to bring you into range.

Table 3.5 lists the most common medications for high cholesterol.

Cholesterol Medications		
Drug Class	**Name of Drug Generic name (Brand)**	**How the drug reacts in the body**
Statins available in the U.S. include:		Inhibit cholesterol synthesis by blocking the enzyme HMG-CoA
	Atorvastatin (Lipitor®)	
	Fluvastatin (Lescol®)	
	Pitavastatin (Livalo®)	
	Lovastatin (Mevacor®, Altoprev™)	
	Pravastatin (Pravachol®)	
	Rosuvastatin Calcium (Crestor®)	
	Simvastatin (Zocor®)	
Statin Combination products:		
	Lovastatin/niacin extended-release (Advicor®)	
	Simvastatin/niacin extendedrelease (Simcor®)	
	Simvastatin/ezetimibe (Vytorin®)	

Continued on following page.

Cholesterol absorption inhibitors	Ezetimibe (Zetia®)	Prevents cholesterol from being absorbed in the intestine. It is the most commonly used nonstatin agent.
Bile acid sequestrants (Available in the U.S.)		Also called bile acid-binding agents, cause the intestine to get rid of more cholesterol.
	Cholestyramine (Questran®, Questran® Light, Prevalite®, Locholest®, Locholest® Light)	
	Colestipol (Colestid®)	
	Colesevelam Hcl (WelChol®)	
PCSK9 inhibitors		
	Alirocumab (Praluent®)	Lowers LDL by Increasing LDL clearance in the body
	Evolocumab (Repatha®)	
Adenosine Triphosphatecitrate Lyase (ACLY)		Works in liver to block the production of cholesterol
	Bempedoic acid (Nexletol®)	
ACLY combination product		
	Bempedoic acid and ezedtimibe (Nexlizet®)	

Continued on following page.

Omega-3 fatty acid ethyl esters (Available in U.S.)		Decrease triglycerides in the blood
	Lovaza®	
	Vascepa™	
	Epanova®	
	Omtryg®	
Fibrates (Available in U.S.)		Decrease triglycerides in the blood
	Gemfibrozil (Lopid®)	
	Fenofibrate (Antara®, Lofibra®, Tricor®, and Triglide™)	
	Fenofibric Acid (Fibricor® and Trilipix®)	

Low Blood Sugar/Hypoglycemia

Low blood sugar or a low glucose level is called **hypogly-cemia**. This condition can occur in people with diabetes for a number of reasons, including taking too much insulin or other medications that lower blood sugar relative to the amount of food eaten. Anyone using insulin or a drug that increases insulin secretion from the pancreas is at risk of hypoglycemia. At first it may seem strange that a person with diabetes, who is usually concerned with controlling high glucose levels in their blood, also needs to be concerned about hypoglycemia. But when you consider the delicate balance you are trying to achieve between good glucose control, insulin, medication and the food you eat, you can see why this is a topic you need to be knowledgeable about.

The ADA consensus statement suggests that any blood glucose level of less than 70 mg/dl (less than 4mmol/L [millimoles per liter; a scientific measurement]) should be considered hypoglycemia. The European Medical Advisory Agency has used 54 mg/dl (3 mmol/L) to define hypoglycemia. Because of these variations in what medical professionals consider the threshold for hypoglycemia, it is important that you work with your physician to determine the glucose level reading that would be considered low for you.

How Glucose Works in Your Body

Between meals, blood glucose levels in your body are maintained by the liver, which produces glucose. The liver produces glucose by the breakdown of **glycogen**. Glycogen is a storage form of excess glucose from the food you eat.

Therefore, glycogen is being replenished each time you eat. During a meal, the body releases insulin in response to the glucose in food and, at the same time, insulin acts on the liver to stop glucose production, because the body's glucose needs are being met through the intake of food. This allows the liver to make more glycogen for later use from the glucose in the food eaten.

Typically, the liver has enough glycogen to make glucose for the first 12 to 24 hours of fasting (no food). The actual length of time is dependent on the amount of glycogen stored and the amount of glucose being used by muscle and fat during that time. As fasting continues and glycogen stored is used up, the kidneys will start to produce glucose, but only in small quantities. After this, the body will start to break down fat and muscle in its search for alternate energy sources. The breakdown of muscle and fat can occur during long periods of fasting, but also occurs in individuals with type 1 diabetes who are not producing insulin and thus glucose is not able to enter the cells, which causes the body to starve. Therefore, a person with type 1 will start to use fat for an energy source because the glucose is not entering the cells as an energy source. That is why individuals with type 1 are very slender or even skinny at diagnosis. When insulin therapy is started, their body is then able to regain its normal weight.

When blood glucose levels become very low, your body will sense the imminent danger and will release stimulating hormones, such as epinephrine (adrenaline) and norepinephrine (noradrenaline), as these hormones will increase glucose levels by initiating glucagon release from the alpha cells of the pancreas. As we learned above, glucagon release from the pancreas stimulates the liver to produce glucose from glycogen, raising blood glucose levels.

For people with type 1 where the beta cells of the pancreas no longer function or with type 2 who have progressed to the point where insulin is no longer produced, the mechanisms described above will no longer occur; the body will have little to no protection against low glucose levels. This is because the ability to suppress insulin and increase glucose can only take place if both insulin and glucagon are produced in your body.

Interesting Fact

A recent study showed that the liver's net glucose production in healthy males was about 1.8 mg/kg per minute during a fast lasting up to 40 hours. That is about ½ an ounce an hour of glucose for a 170-pound person.

Healthy adults need an estimated 1 mg/kg of glucose per minute to keep adequate brain function. That is 100 grams a day for a 154-pound person.

Why Low Glucose Levels Are Dangerous

Your brain utilizes glucose for fuel. It cannot make glucose or store more than a few minutes' worth of glycogen supply. An inadequate glucose supply to the brain results in brain dysfunction that, if prolonged, will cause irreversible nerve damage. Therefore, the brain needs a constant supply of glucose to keep functioning. When blood glucose levels get low, there are a number of mechanisms that go into action to help provide glucose until an outside source brings the level back to normal. The risk in this process is that when the other glucose sources are used up you are in danger of losing consciousness, going into a coma, or even dying.

When glucose levels become low, the brain's ability to function correctly is impaired. The first signs are usually behavioral changes, such as feeling tired, irritated, or anxious. As glucose levels continue to decrease, confusion and tiredness set in. At this point, the situation may become particularly critical. You may not be able to help yourself because your brain is not able to process and function properly anymore. The scary part of this scenario is that the process can be so gradual that you do not even realize anything is happening until it is too late and you pass out. That is why frequent blood glucose testing will help you know if your glucose levels are low, even if you do not yet have any of the symptoms just described.

The symptoms of low blood sugar are:
- Shakiness, anxiety, nervousness
- Sweating
- Irritability and other behavior changes; crying, feeling weak
- Confusion
- Restlessness at night
- Impatience
- Chills and clamminess
- Rapid heart beat
- Passing out; loss of consciousness

What To Do When You Are Experiencing Low Blood Sugar

Glucose is a simple sugar (carbohydrate), as opposed to the complex sugars found in fruit, vegetables, nuts, seeds, and grains. Since the brain can only utilize simple sugar (glucose) to function, if your glucose reading is low, it is imperative that you replenish your body with simple sugar; for example, sugar, honey, glucose tablets, etc., that can have an effect on the brain right away. Proteins or fats will have no effect on providing glucose to the brain. Complex sugars will take too long to break down into simple sugars and be delivered to the brain.

Therefore, simple sugar is king for lows, but you need to know how much to ingest to reestablish normal brain function and bring balance back to your body. Here is a typical action plan: If you test low, drink or eat 15 to 20 grams of simple sugar, wait 15 minutes, then retest your blood glucose. If you are still low, take another 15 to 20 grams of simple sugar, wait 15 minutes again and retest.

The following chart shows some easy ways to ingest these amounts in a hurry.

Skittles	1 Skittle = 1 gram of sugar
Soda	1 ounce = 3 grams of sugar (one 12-ounce can has about 36 grams of sugar; half a can has about 13 grams of sugar)
Sugar	1 teaspoon = 4 grams of sugar
Honey	1 teaspoon = 5 grams of sugar
Lifesavers	1 Lifesaver = 2.5 grams of sugar
Glucose tablet	1 tablet = 4 grams of sugar

Typically, your blood glucose level will have returned to normal at this point; if it has not, you should call your physician. Once your blood glucose has returned to a safe level, a well-balanced snack, such as a sandwich, is a good choice to stabilize your glucose level. You need to eat a well-balanced snack because simple sugar is metabolized (used for energy) by the body very quickly and is used up just as fast.

If blood glucose gets too low, the brain will not function at a level in which you can take care of yourself. Signs of this would be an inability to answer questions, being unable to eat or drink, being unconscious, and/or having seizures. Your physician may prescribe a glucagon injection that comes in a glucagon kit, which can be given while awaiting medical assistance. Glucagon acts only on liver glycogen to produce glucose. If you are given a glucagon kit, it is important to open it, read the directions and do a practice drill so that there will be no delays in an emergency situation. You and your physician should work together to determine when to administer a glucagon shot.

How to Prevent Hypoglycemia

The best way to try and prevent low blood sugar is to have both a daily and an emergency action plan that you develop with your physician.

A daily action plan should include:

- The minimum number of times a day you should test, as well as the times of day to test

- A step-by-step plan for what to do if the test result is too high or low

- Always carry emergency sugar with you to use if your blood glucose gets low, as well as a healthy snack to eat after you stabilize your glucose level

- Make sure you have enough test strips with you to test throughout the day

- Test before driving

- Program your phone with important numbers in case you are not feeling well

- Make sure your family, friends and co-workers know the signs of low blood glucose so they can check on you and help you if necessary

- If you are planning to do strenuous exercise or start a team sport, carry extra snacks. At the end of your workout, remember that even when you are done, your muscles are still active and are metabolizing glucose, which can cause a low glucose reading several hours later, so test frequently. Exercise also increases insulin sensitivity, allowing glucose to be used more efficiently. This effect can last up to 24 hours after exercise.

- Of note: Alcohol inhibits glucose production in the body. Therefore, if you ingest a significant amount of alcohol in the evening, then essentially fast (no food) during your night of sleep, you run an increased risk of hypoglycemia the following morning.

An emergency action plan should include:

- Your full and detailed action plan placed where everyone can see and find it

- A glucagon injection kit kept in a permanent location; train your family, friends, and co-workers on when and how to use it, including how much to give and how long to wait to see if it has worked

- The glucose level determined by you and your physician that signifies you are out of danger

- Make sure your plan is clear that no liquids should be given if you are unconscious

- When to call 911

You and your physician should develop your emergency action plan together and you should practice it at least once or twice with your family, friends, and co-workers. Why? Because the middle of a real emergency is not the time to be reading the instructions on how to give a glucagon shot for the first time!

Summary

Awareness of high blood pressure, high cholesterol and low blood sugar is essential to prevent complications.

All three conditions have a silent period. You may be in danger and be totally unaware of what is happening unless you get regular tests.

- Blood pressure is known as the <u>silent killer</u> because there may not be any signs that it is out of control. You can avoid this if you regularly monitor your blood pressure.

- High cholesterol can cause <u>silent ischemia,</u> which can lead to heart attacks and stroke. This may not happen if you monitor your cholesterol.

- Low blood glucose can slowly or rapidly occur <u>without noticeable signs</u>. By the time symptoms are apparent you may not be able to take care of yourself, which can lead to unconsciousness or worse.

Reading these chapters and becoming aware of how complications develop gives you a big edge on how to keep healthy and why you need to do it. My son has been vigilant about controlling his diabetes since he was diagnosed. I often tell him that, even though he has diabetes, he will be healthier than many of his friends when they are all in their 40s because he has been constantly monitoring his health. He exercises regularly and will be physically fit. He will have better weight control because of the healthy food he eats, and he will have more energy, vitality and good looks than friends who do not have diabetes and have not been living a healthy lifestyle. So, I think that if having diabetes helps you to stay as attractive and fit in your 40s as you were in your 20s, then you have learned one of the secrets of living an optimal life.

Facts at a Glance

1. Blood Pressure

Getting your blood pressure under control is probably the <u>greatest protection</u> you have to prevent stroke, as well as kidney, heart and eye damage.

2. Heart Problems and Cholesterol

There are several reasons why cholesterol build up may occur, such as diet, a genetic predisposition, or a combination of both. Eating a well-balanced diet to control your weight and overall health is an important consideration.

3. Low Blood Sugar

Testing with a blood glucose machine (glucometer) daily and when you have symptoms of low blood sugar will help prevent extreme low glucose. <u>Severe</u> low blood sugar requires an emergency action plan. This is something you need to develop with your physician <u>before</u> there is an emergency.

Be prepared for low blood sugar by keeping a few snacks on hand that will provide you with simple sugars, such as Skittles, soda (like Coke), honey, sugar, glucose tablets, or Lifesavers. This will help you quickly reverse low blood sugar.

Your Three Action Steps

1. Ask your physician if your blood pressure is at goal for someone with diabetes. If not, create an action plan with your physician using exercise and medication. (See Figure 3.3 on pages 79-80 for a list of common medications to treat high blood pressure.)

2. Ask your physician if your cholesterol is in control. If not, create an action plan with exercise and medication. (See Table 3.4 on pages 81-86 for a list of medications commonly used to treat high cholesterol.)

3. Know the signs and symptoms of low blood sugar and create a low blood sugar action plan with your physician.

Chapter 4

How Do I Prevent Complications of Kidney, Eye, and Nerve Damage?

Introduction

This chapter dives right into the complications that may arise by exposing your body to hyperglycemia over a long period of time. Your risk of chronic complications is associated with having constant high blood glucose for many years, but the good news is that you can lower your risk.

Two landmark studies, the Diabetes Control and Complications Trial (DCCT) and United Kingdom Prospective Diabetes Study (UKPDS) both showed that, in individuals with type 1 or type 2 diabetes, a 1 percent decrease in A1C reduces the risk of microvascular complications by approximately 30 percent. In fact, the UKPDS study of type 2 diabetes showed that just a 0.9 percent difference in A1C levels (a median A1C of 7.0 percent versus a median A1C of 7.9 percent), resulted in a significant reduction in microvascular complications.

Another study, called the Epidemiology of Diabetes Interventions and Complications (EDIC), showed that people with type 1 diabetes who had early intensive glycemic control for 6.5 years had a significant reduction in cardiovascular complications during a mean follow up of 17 years. The EDIC study also pointed out that the benefits of early intervention with intense treatment are only seen after many years.

Chronic complications that arise with diabetes can be divided into two groups called macrovascular and microvascular. Macrovascular means large blood vessels (macro = large, vascular = blood vessels). Macrovascular complications include heart disease called coronary artery disease, brain or stroke complications called cerebrovascular disease, and narrowing of arteries in the lower part of the body called peripheral arterial disease.

Microvascular is a term that means small blood vessel (micro = small, vascular = blood vessels). Microvascular complications include kidney disease called nephropathy, eye disease called retinopathy, and nerve damage disease called neuropathy. Microvascular complications in both type 1 and type 2 diabetes are the result of chronic hyperglycemia. Large studies have conclusively demonstrated that a reduction in chronic high blood glucose prevents or delays retinopathy, neuropathy, and nephropathy.

In this section, we will look at microvascular complications; kidney, eye, and nerve disease; and will finish up with a saying or acronym that provides you with a way to remember the yearly tests necessary to help you stay in control of your diabetes.

Not long ago, I was vacationing in Hawaii when I ran into a former neighbor whom I had not seen in about seven years. I will refer to him as Mr. Smith. He was enjoying paradise in Hawaii with his family and we had the opportunity to spend some time catching up. Needless to say, the conversation moved to the topic of health and I found out that Mr. Smith had been diagnosed with diabetes several years before. Moreover, he had just recently been released from a hospital stay brought on by diabetes and other complications. Of course I had a lot to say on the subject.

Perhaps you can imagine my surprise, though, when we sat down at the poolside café where a hamburger and a drink were waiting for Mr. Smith, compliments of his wife. Mr. Smith ate his hamburger. I knew he did not test before he ate, because I was with him the whole time.

I said, "Did you test your glucose before your meal?"

He answered no.

"Okay, what type of medication are you on?"

"Insulin."

I slowly said, "Okaaayyy...," but it was the only word I spoke slowly because I needed to give Mr. Smith as much information about diabetes as I could right away in case he decided never to talk to me again!

The scary part of this conversation was that Mr. Smith did not have a good understanding of how insulin worked or how fast his particular insulin worked. He was unaware of why it was important to test his blood glucose or what other medications should be prescribed, but he did not have an action plan for his health.

I am happy to say that Mr. Smith was gracious enough to allow me to spend two hours with him going over diabetes treatment. We learned that Mr. Smith's physician had not given him enough education about his diabetes, information that could have relieved many troublesome days of not feeling well and possibly have prevented his hospitalization. If only Mr. Smith had even a little knowledge of diabetes, he could have asked some pertinent questions, which could have opened a real line of communication with his physician.

About a month after I returned home, I received a lovely letter from Mr. Smith thanking me for the information I had given him. Most importantly, he told me that he now works closely with his endocrinologist to control his blood sugar and is feeling 100% better. In his own words: "Good morning, Christine. Yesterday's visit with my endocrinologist was a great success. He said the list of questions given to him in Hawaii was excellent and carefully answered each one."

Wow! Think about Mr. Smith's situation! Two hours of education out of about seven years of disease possibly saved his life, and definitely gave him the ability to feel better and live life more fully. Are two to three hours of diabetes education worth a lifetime of feeling better so you can live an optimal life? I hope you will agree that they are!

I trust this chapter will motivate you to test your blood sugar at home more frequently. As you learned in an earlier chapter, there is a relationship between blood glucose results and A1C results. If your home blood glucose is continually high, your A1C will be high too. Do not wait for your next appointment to talk to your physician. Call and make an appointment today and work with your physician to get your blood glucose within your goal range.

Diabetic Nephropathy (Kidney Disease)

Diabetic nephropathy is a condition that occurs when the kidneys of a person with diabetes are not functioning correctly, which is shown by protein in the urine. Protein in the urine is an early warning sign of kidney problems. The extent of kidney damage can be estimated by a test called the glomerular filtration rate (GFR), which calculates how much blood each minute passes through the tiny filters in the kidneys, called glomeruli. Your GFR depends on your age, gender, race, and the amount of creatinine in your blood. Creatinine is a waste material produced by using the muscles in your body and is removed by the kidneys. The better your kidneys are functioning, the lower your blood serum creatinine levels will be and the higher your GFR will be. Ideally, your glomerular filtration rate should be above 90.

You probably know that your kidneys produce urine, but do you know all the other functions your kidneys perform?

Your kidneys:

- help regulate blood pressure, which is important to the health of all the other organs in your body

- increase red blood cell production so you have enough to carry oxygen throughout your body

- regulate calcium for strong bones and teeth

- are involved in vitamin D activation so calcium can be absorbed

- filter toxic substances in your blood to protect the body from being poisoned

- eliminate excess water from the body, which decreases extra pressure on your heart

- and keep the delicate acid base (pH) balance in

check that is vital to all the processes in the body.

Amazing! And these are just the main functions. I consider the kidneys to be one of the greatest regulator organs in the body.

Your kidneys are located near the middle of your back on either side of your spine and weigh about 5 ounces each. These fist-sized powerhouses are a very important filtering system that process about 200 quarts of blood a day and sift out about two quarts of waste products and extra water to be excreted as urine. Wastes in the blood come from the normal breakdown of active tissues, such as muscles, and from food. After the body has taken what it needs from food for energy and repairs, wastes are sent to the blood to be removed by the kidneys. When your kidneys are not working well, wastes and fluid affect all the organs in your body, so it is especially important to protect them.

Diabetic kidney disease or nephropathy (nephro = kidney, pathy = disease) is the most common cause of endstage renal (kidney) disease in the United States and diabetes is the leading cause of chronic kidney disease. The United States Renal Data System shows that diabetes accounts for 45% of all kidney failures. People with type 1 or type 2 diabetes are both at risk.

Twenty to 30 percent of people with diabetes will show signs of kidney disease after having diabetes for approximately 15 years. With type 1, it is clear when diabetes started; therefore, we know that 20 to 30 percent develop kidney disease somewhere between 10 and 15 years after diagnosis. Individuals who do not demonstrate kidney disease within 20 to 25 years post-diabetes diagnosis then have very little chance (approximately 1 percent) of developing nephropathy. This statistic is a powerful reminder to keep your blood glucose and blood pressure under control.

In type 2, however, the individual may have already had the disease for years before being diagnosed. According to the United Kingdom Prospective Diabetes Study (UKPDS), the development of kidney disease in people with type 2 diabetes within ten years of diagnosis is 25 percent, but 5 percent of those diagnosed will have great kidney damage. With the current rise in type 2 diabetes mellitus, rates of diabetic kidney disease are projected to continue to increase over the next two decades, with African-American and Native American males at higher risk than other groups.

Kidney Function

Your kidneys have about a million tiny units within them called nephrons, each of which is capable of forming urine. The kidneys cannot regenerate (make new) nephrons. Each nephron has two major components:

1. a glomerulus - a delicate network of blood vessels or capillaries through which large amounts of fluid are filtered from the blood and

2. a long tubule that converts the filtered fluid into urine.

Urine formation begins with large amounts of fluid being filtered by the blood vessels in the glomerulus called glomerular capillaries. The glomerulus acts as a filtering unit, keeping normal proteins and cells in the bloodstream, and allowing extra fluid and wastes to pass through into the urine. The fluid that is allowed to be filtered does not contain protein. This filtered fluid from the glomerulus now goes through a long tube called a tubule. The tubules evaluate the filtered fluid and see what substances should be excreted in the urine and what should be reabsorbed into the body.

There are three ways the substances in the fluid are handled in the tubules:

1. The substance can be allowed to go straight into urine. Waste products from your muscles, called creatinine, are handled in this manner.

2. The substance can be passed into urine, but how much is passed is adjusted according to your body's needs, such as electrolytes, sodium, potassium, etc.

3. The substances, such as protein or albumin and glucose, can be reabsorbed back into the blood, not passing any of it into the urine.

If your kidneys are not functioning correctly and these wastes are not removed, they will build up in your blood and damage other organs. Over a long period of time, this causes other chronic complications and slowly poisons the body. If excess fluid is not removed it causes your heart to work harder, which in turn may increase blood pressure, as well as creating a feeling of discomfort similar to when one is bloated.

Pathogenesis – How Diabetic Kidney Disease (Nephropathy) Develops

Diabetic nephropathy is a condition that is caused by hyperglycemia (high blood glucose), hypertension (high blood pressure), and protein in the urine called proteinuria.

It is a combination of these three conditions that activates processes in the body that hurt the kidneys. The network of blood vessels in the glomerulus in the kidneys is very sensitive to change; changes in blood pressure and high levels of blood glucose injure the tiny capillaries in the kidney glomerulus and surrounding tissues.

High Blood Sugar

High blood sugar is thought to directly injure the tiny capillaries called glomerulus because glucose reacts with the glomerular tissues. When glucose attaches to tissue proteins or free amino acids that are circulating through the blood, it produces a substance called advanced glycosylated end products (AGEs). Once the AGEs are formed, the reaction is not reversible and they gradually build up over the lifetime of the protein. The buildup of AGEs cross-links with tissues, causing kidney's glomerulus to dysfunction. The serum levels of the AGEs correlate with the level of high blood glucose, and as AGEs build up, glomerular filtration rate (GFR) declines. This phenomenon is specific to people with diabetes and does not occur in normal kidneys. AGEs directly alter the structure and function of the kidneys. Early glucose reaction with kidney proteins is reversible, but later AGEs are irreversible.

High glucose also causes damage by supporting the formation of sorbitol. The cells of the kidneys allow free interchange of glucose in and out of the cell; these cells will use glucose for energy. Excess glucose that is not used for energy can enter a metabolic pathway called the polyol pathway and be converted to sorbitol. Sorbitol cannot cross the cell membrane, and it builds up, causing osmotic pressure on the cell by dragging water into the cells and promoting cell damage. High sorbitol levels can also increase substances, such as reactive oxygen, that cause future cell damage, and can injure the kidneys by becoming oxidized to fructose which is another type of sugar, and can lead to more AGE production. The vicious cycle continues when glucose blood levels are not controlled.

High Blood Pressure

High blood pressure can damage the glomeruli and blood vessels of your kidneys by putting extra stress or force on the blood vessels, destroying them and preventing the kidneys from filtering the blood as they are supposed to. Abnormal kidney function can cause further increases in high blood pressure, resulting in a destructive cycle. The development of protein in the urine is usually equal to the rise in systemic blood pressure, and there is a significant correlation between the rate of decline in glomerular filtration and the blood pressure levels. Likewise, a decrease in blood pressure has been shown to protect the kidneys and decrease protein in the urine.

High blood pressure interferes with regulation of the kidneys' glomerular capillary pressure, which is vital to normal filtration and urine formation. The pressure in the glomerular capillaries is tightly regulated by precise adjustments of two arteries called the afferent and efferent arteries. The afferent (artery going to the kidney) and efferent (artery going away from the kidney) are very sensitive to pressure. High blood glucose can cause a significant reduction in afferent and efferent arteriolar pressure. This causes an increase in glomerular capillary pressure added on top of blood pressure. All of this causes further kidney damage.

Proteinuria

Protein in the urine is a strong and independent predictor of decline in kidney function. Excess protein appears to cause damage to the tubules in the kidneys and contributes to the progression of kidney disease.

Symptoms of Chronic Kidney Disease That Lead to Diabetic Nephropathy

People in the early stages of chronic kidney disease (CKD) causing diabetic nephropathy usually do not feel sick at all and have no symptoms.

People with worsening kidney disease may:

- need to urinate more often or less often

- feel tired

- lose their appetite, or experience nausea and vomiting

- have swelling in their hands or feet

- feel itchy or numb

- get drowsy or have trouble concentrating

- have darkened skin
- have muscle cramps

Diagnosing Diabetic Nephropathy

Albuminuria

Diabetic nephropathy is diagnosed by screening for the presence of a protein called albumin in the urine, and screening for a buildup of creatinine and urea nitrogen in the blood. When albumin is found in your urine, it signifies that the glomerulus is not working well. Remember, there should be no protein in your urine. A diagnosis of albuminuria is given when small or large amounts of albumin are found in the urine. The more albumin found in your urine, the worse the kidney disease. Table 4.1 shows the diagnostic ranges for this test.

Definition of the Severity of Albumin (Protein) in the Urine < means less than > means greater than		
Category	Spot Collection in ug/g	Results
Albuminuria	< 30	Normal
Albuminuria	30 - 300	Beginning of damage
Albuminuria	>300	Damage is certain
Albuminuria	>3,500	Severe damage

Table 4.1 Diagnostic ranges for albumin in urine

If your first laboratory test shows high levels of albumin, you should have another test done one to two weeks later to confirm the results.

Glomerular Filtration Rate (GFR)

If you have taken two tests for albuminuria and both tests show higher than normal results, it is called persistent proteinuria and indicates some level of kidney disease. Your physician will want to determine your exact level of kidney function and assess what stage of disease you have. This can be done by calculating your glomerular filtration rate (GFR) using your serum creatinine measurements, and factoring in your age, race, sex, and other factors to arrive at a value.

Table 4.2 shows the diagnostic ranges and classifications for glomerular filtration rate (GFR) testing.

Chronic Kidney Disease Classification Based on Glomerular Filtration Rate (GFR) (ml/min/1.73m^2		
Stage 1	Normal to high	$\geq$90
Stage 2	Mildly decreased	60-89
Stage 3a	Mild to moderate decrease	45-59
Stage 3b	Moderately to severely decreased	30-44
Stage 4	Severely decreased	15-29
Stage 5	Kidney failure	<15

Table 4.2 Classification of kidney disease

Serum Creatinine

Serum creatinine is another waste product in the blood created by the normal breakdown of muscle cells during activity. Healthy kidneys take creatinine out of the blood and put it into the urine to leave the body. If your kidneys are not working well, creatinine will build up in the blood, so a blood screening for the presence of elevated creatinine levels can also help determine the presence and severity of kidney damage. Your doctor can use the results of your creatinine test to determine the extent of kidney damage by using your glomerular filtration rate, or GFR.

Individuals who are at high risk, such as those with diabetes or high blood pressure, should also have the albumin-to-creatinine measurement to detect kidney disease.

When to Begin Testing for Diabetic Nephropathy

Because diabetic kidney disease affects up to 35 percent of people with type 1 diabetes and 30 to 40 percent of people with type 2, screening for chronic kidney disease should begin five years after the diagnosis of type 1 diabetes and at the time of diagnosis of type 2 diabetes.

Type 1 individuals with kidney disease almost always have other diabetic microvascular complications, such as eye and nerve disease. In type 2 diabetes, eye disease is less likely to happen with about 40% lacking retinopathy.

Prevention and Treatment

The optimal treatment for diabetic nephropathy is to prevent it with good blood glucose control. Performing your tests on schedule so that you always know your numbers is equally important. Albuminuria should be tested as early as possible after diagnosis if you have type 2 diabetes, as well as every year, along with a measurement of your serum creatinine so that your physician can estimate your glomerular filtration rate.

If you have been diagnosed with kidney disease and high blood pressure, you can slow down its progression by controlling your blood glucose and by controlling your blood pressure by taking a medication called an angiotensin-converting enzyme inhibitor (ACE) or angiotensin II receptor blocker (ARB) medication if your doctor recommends it. These medicines may prevent or stop kidney damage if caught early. The ADA recommends checking your blood pressure at every routine diabetes test visit, and keeping blood pressure below 130/80. If you are diagnosed with type 2 diabetes and diabetic kidney disease with normal blood pressure, the ADA recommends different medications in a class called sodium-glucose cotransport 2 inhibitor or glucagon-like peptide 1 agonist. Two examples in each class would be Jardiance and Farxiga or Trulicity or Victoza.

Experts disagree about how much protein people with diabetes and kidney disease should eat, but evidence shows that too much or too little protein can be harmful. The ADA recommends approximately 0.8 g/kg per day. This can vary depending upon what your physician feels is the best for you.

Stop smoking. In addition to increasing your risk of a heart attack and stroke, smoking speeds up the progression of kidney disease.

If you are overweight, try to lose weight. Being overweight contributes to kidney disease by making diabetes harder to control, raising blood pressure, blood glucose, and causing scarring in the kidneys. In a small study of overweight patients with chronic protein in the urine, the amount of protein was significantly decreased at five months among dieters who lost on average 4 percent of their body weight.

Diabetic nephropathy is, unfortunately, an all-too-common complication of diabetes. While there are certain risk factors, such as a family history of kidney disease, or being African American, Hispanic, or Native American, there is also good evidence that early detection and treatment prevents the onset of the disease. Again, getting control of your blood glucose levels, and getting all of your tests done regularly will help protect you against this complication.

Diabetic Retinopathy (Eye Disease)

The encouraging news is that diabetic retinopathy (retino = retina of the eye, pathy = disease) is preventable with good glucose control. You do not need to have eye problems when you are diligent about your diabetes. However, this disease poses a serious risk, as people with diabetes are 25 times more likely to become legally blind than individuals who do not have diabetes. The longer you have had diabetes without controlling your blood sugar, the greater the possibility you will develop eye disease.

In individuals with type 1 diabetes, 23 percent will develop diabetic eye disease or retinopathy within five years of diagnosis. Therefore, people with type 1 diabetes should have their first dilated and comprehensive eye exam within 5 years after diagnosis. After 10 to 15 years of having diabetes, the percentage increases.

For people with type 2 diabetes, 20 percent will already show some form of eye disease at the time they are diagnosed, which will increase after 15 years. People with type 2 are more likely to have diabetic retinopathy at the time they are diagnosed and are more likely to develop diabetic retinopathy sooner after diagnosis than patients with type 1. This is because individuals with type 2 often have no symptoms of diabetes for a long time and do not seek medical help. Two studies called The Diabetes Control and Complication Trial (DCCT) and the United Kingdom Prospective Diabetes Study (UKPDS) have documented that good glucose control can decrease the risk of diabetic retinopathy. Early detection and treatment are essential, but it is estimated that only 55 percent of people with diabetes receive adequate eye care.

What is Diabetic Retinopathy?

The retina of your eye is a transparent light-sensing neural tissue with a rich blood supply. The retina covers the inside of the back of your eye, which is called the fundus. This is why retinal eye examination is called fundoscopy. In normal vision, light rays enter the eye through the pupil and pass through the lens and vitreous gel until they reach the retina. The retina contains photoreceptors (light receptors) that change light into nerve signals that are sent by the optic nerve to the brain. The macula at the center of the retina contains the most photoreceptors. The fovea at the center of the macula processes the details needed for reading and driving. Damage to the macula is vision threatening.

Figure 4.3 shows the anatomy of the eye.

Figure 4.3 Anatomy of the eye.

Available at www.nei.nih.gov/photo/charts/index.asp. From National Eye Institutes of Health

Diabetic retinopathy can cause vision loss by three mechanisms:

1. lack of oxygen in the macula called macular ischemia

2. bleeding called hemorrhage

3. or retinal detachment.

This damage will occur within or on the retina. Neural photoreceptor damage may occur before blood vessel damage, causing altered color perception and contrast. Then as diabetic retinopathy progresses, blood vessel damage occurs leading to a buildup of fluid called diabetic macular edema or (DME), vascular wall distortion, called non-proliferative diabetic retinopathy or (NPDR), and neovascularization, called proliferative diabetic retinopathy or (PDR).

High blood glucose in diabetes destroys the cells that maintain the structural strength of the retinal capillaries, resulting in weakened out-pouching of these tiny blood vessels, called microaneurysms that can and do leak. Microaneurysms are the earliest visible sign of vascular wall distortion in the eye and looks like small red dots within the retina. If the microaneurysms leak and the fluid builds up between the layers of the retina, it can cause inadequate oxygen supply or referred to as ischemia. Significant fluid leakage in the macula can cause temporary or permanent vision loss. Fluid in the macula may occur at any stage in the progression of diabetic retinopathy; if it is not treated promptly, macular ischemia may destroy the photoreceptors resulting in permanent loss of vision.

As diabetic retinopathy progresses, your body will compensate for the lack of oxygen (worsening ischemia) by forming new blood vessels in the eye. This process is called neovascularization and occurs on the surface of the retina to bring oxygen to those tissues. However, these fragile new vessels will attach themselves to other blood vessels; normal body motion can cause them to shear off and bleed, causing sudden temporary vision loss. Fibrous tissue may then form near and on the damaged vessel. Over time, as the tissue contracts, it pulls the retina from the sclera, causing vision loss.

Pathogenesis – How Diabetic Retinopathy Develops

The reason individuals with diabetes develop eye disease is due to high blood glucose levels, which result in damage to the structure and function of the retinal capillaries. When these capillaries are damaged there is an increase in capillary leakage and edema (swelling). The capillaries lose their elasticity and can no longer accommodate changes in blood pressure. Capillary vascular tone is decreased by high glucose, resulting in increased eye blood pressure. There is also increased thickening of the blood vessels, which decreases the availability of oxygen, leading to ischemia. Because capillary damage alters retinal blood flow, the body starts to form new blood retinal capillaries to compensate.

Some of the mechanisms of high blood glucose that destroy the retinal capillaries are believed to be the same for all diabetic small vascular complications, including kidney and nerve damage. The same mechanisms of damage that occur in the capillary vessels of the kidneys also occur in the eyes:

- High blood glucose can bond to proteins and produce advanced glycosylation end products (AGEs). These AGEs can cross-link to proteins in the capillaries and cause capillary cellular dysfunction and destruction.

- High blood glucose can lead to glucose being metabolized to sorbitol. Sorbitol cannot cross cell membranes and begins to build up. The excess sorbitol drags water into the cell, causing cellular stress that eventually leads to destruction.

- Protein kinase C (an enzyme that controls the function of other proteins) increases with high blood glucose levels, which results in cell damage and dysfunction.

Symptoms of Diabetic Retinopathy

It is possible to have diabetic retinopathy for a long time and not notice any symptoms. At the point that you are noticing symptoms, significant damage has already occurred.

Symptoms of diabetic retinopathy and its complications may include:
- Blurred or distorted vision, or difficulty reading
- Floaters (shadows, dark specks, strings, or cobwebs that "float" across your vision)
- Partial or total loss of vision, or a shadow or veil across your field of vision
- Pain in the eye

Diagnosing Diabetic Retinopathy

You will need to see an ophthalmologist (eye doctor) or optometrist for your yearly dilated eye exam. This is the only way to check to see if you have diabetic retinopathy. This exam cannot be performed by your primary care doctor, as your pupils must be dilated in order to do a comprehensive examination. When you visit an ophthal-mologist or optometrist, some of the tests that may be per-formed include the following

- A visual acuity test. This measures the eye's abil-ity to focus and see details at both near and far distances.

- A comprehensive dilated eye exam. Drops will be placed in your eyes to widen or dilate your pupils to allow your doctor a better view inside your eyes.

- Ophthalmoscopy and slit lamp exam. These two tests allow a view of the back of your eye and other structures within your eye. This is where your eye doctor can detect any signs of diabetic retinopathy. Some of the signs include microaneurysms, neovas-cularization and cotton wool spots.

- Fluorescein angiography is a test where a dye is injected into a vein in your arm. Then pictures are taken as the dye circulates through your eyes' blood vessels. This test can tell if the blood vessels are closed, broken, or leaking.

- Optical coherence tomography (OCT) is a test that takes cross-sectional pictures of the retina. This will tell the physician how much fluid if any leaked into the retina. This test can also monitor how well the treatment plan is working.

When to Begin Testing

If you have not been diagnosed with diabetic retinopathy, the ADA recommends the following screening guidelines:

- People with type 1 diabetes who are 10 years of age and older should have a dilated eye examination within five years of being diagnosed and every year after that.

- People with type 2 diabetes should have a dilated eye exam as soon as diabetes is diagnosed and every year after that.

- Women with either type 1 or type 2 diabetes who are considering pregnancy should have an examination before becoming pregnant.

Prevention and Treatment

Because retinopathy is a microvascular complication of diabetes, it is essential to have yearly dilated eye exams because damage in your eyes can go unnoticed until there is a decrease or loss of vision, at which point the disease has already progressed. The sobering fact about retinopathy is that once it has advanced, improved glucose control shows less benefit than if blood glucose had been controlled in the early stages. This is exactly why it is so important for good glucose control early on, prompt detection of any problems, and timely blood pressure control. The Wisconsin Epidemiologic Study of Diabetic Retinopathy (WESDR) and other studies have shown a direct correlation between A1C levels and the severity of diabetic retinopathy. The Diabetes Control and Complication Trial (DCCT) and United Kingdom Prospective Diabetes Study (UKPDS) established that intense glucose control reduced the incidence and progression of diabetic retinopathy in both type 1 and type 2 diabetes.

Even if you do not have diabetes, hypertension alone

can cause retinopathy, with many of the same types of damage of diabetic retinopathy. Therefore, blood pressure control is another area that can help decrease or slow down the progression of diabetic retinopathy.

Treatment of diabetic retinopathy consists of laser photocoagulation, which is usually helpful if it is performed before the retina has become severely damaged. Intravitreous injections of antivascular endothelial growth factor are a reasonable alternative to traditional laser photocoagulation. These methods are helpful in treating the symptoms of the disease, but they cannot cure it. People who have received treatments for diabetic retinopathy may need to be monitored more frequently to check for any new changes or progression of the disease.

The ADA recommends the following:

- Stop smoking; smoking increases the risk of diabetic retinopathy

- If you have been diagnosed with diabetic retinopathy, you should be referred to an ophthalmologist (eye doctor) who is knowledgeable and experienced in the management and treatment of diabetic retinopathy.

Diabetic retinopathy is a very serious complication of diabetes, but you can lower your risk by being aggressive about your blood glucose control, as well as keeping your blood pressure and cholesterol levels within normal range.

Diabetic Neuropathy (Nerve Damage)

Diabetic neuropathy (neuro = nerve, pathy = disease) is a condition in which the body's nerves become damaged. The result is a decrease or absence of feeling or sensation of pain in the affected area. If you have diabetes, this needs to be of great concern to you, as diabetic neuropathy occurs in about 50 percent of individuals with longstanding type 1 or type 2 diabetes. It is related to the length of time an individual has had diabetes and how well they have controlled their blood glucose.

Here are some of the risk factors for diabetic neuropathy:

- Age
- Length of time you have had diabetes
- Degree of blood glucose control
- Excess weight (the greater your body mass index [BMI], the greater your risk)
- Elevated cholesterol and triglyceride levels
- Hypertension (high blood pressure)
- Other microvascular complications
- Smoking

There are many different forms of neuropathy, but the most common is lower body nerve damage in your feet, ankles, and legs. This is the form we will discuss, using the term sensory neuropathy to describe the condition.

Pathogenesis – How Sensory Neuropathy Develops

Diabetic neuropathy is a microvascular (small blood vessel) disease, as blood vessels and nerves are closely related and intertwined. Your nerves depend on adequate blood flow for oxygen and blood vessels depend on normal nerve functions to regulate their diameter. Arteries regulate their inner vessel diameter, and thus blood flow, by contracting the surrounding muscular wall. The ability to do this is controlled by the nervous system. With the onset of sensory neuropathy, one of the changes that occurs is narrowing of the blood vessels called vasoconstriction that can lead to blood vessel abnormalities, decreased oxygen tension and lack of adequate oxygen supply to the nerves. Nerve damage caused by decreased oxygen is well established in diabetic neuropathy.

There are several different possible mechanisms that lead to sensory neuropathy, all of which involve high blood glucose levels and all of which are very similar to the conditions associated with kidney and eye disease. They include:

- High blood glucose can bond to proteins and produce advanced glycosylation end products (AGEs). These AGEs may disrupt the integrity and repair of neurons through interference with nerve cell metabolism and nerve transmission.

- High blood glucose can lead to glucose being metabolized to sorbitol. Sorbitol cannot cross cell membranes and accumulates. The sorbitol can be further metabolized to fructose causing reduced nerve myoinositol and decreased nerve transmission.

- Protein kinase C is increased with high blood sugar levels, causing reduced nerve blood flow and decreased nerve conduction, which is important for feeling sensory stimuli.

Symptoms of Sensory Neuropathy

The symptoms of sensory neuropathy may include tingling, numbness, prickling, burning, and stabbing or shooting pain. These sensations can start in your feet and spread up your legs and may increase at nighttime. As nerve damage progresses, the pain may go away, but the loss of feeling and numbness remains.

Sensory nerve damage is usually accompanied by motor (movement) nerve damage, referred to as sensorimotor neuropathy. Motor nerve damage may cause small muscle wasting and loss of reflexes, such as the ankle reflexes. Motor nerve damage symptoms may come and go for years, but gradually tend to improve over time. Unfortunately, this improvement is often followed by progressive sensory or feeling loss, leaving you at risk for foot injuries.

The danger of decreased or loss of sensation in your feet is that you may be unaware that an injury has occurred or that the shoes you are wearing are putting undue pressure on a portion of your foot, thus increasing the chance of a sore. Once there is a cut or any type of break in your skin, there is a possibility of infection. People with diabetes need to be especially concerned about infection, because high glucose levels in your blood and body fluids provide ideal conditions for fungus and bacteria to multiply rapidly. Diabetic foot infections are common, so you need to act fast to clear up any infection before it spreads. Shallow cuts or ulcers can quickly develop into limb-threatening infections requiring amputation. Treatment of infections involves both antibiotic therapy and aggressive maintenance of good blood glucose levels.

Prevention and Control

Individuals with diabetic sensory nerve damage may have no symptoms, so it is important to have a thorough foot examination done yearly at your physician's office, as well as daily foot self-examinations. When you are at your physician's office, your exam should be done with your socks and shoes off. Your doctor should carefully inspect both your feet to see if there are any sores or ulcers, dry skin, cracks, or ingrown toenails. Ankle reflexes should be checked for motor function. A pressure sensation test should be done using the 10-g monofilament pinprick test. The 10-g monofilament test uses a nylon filament or wire mounted in a holder that is designed to deliver 10 grams of force (this is very light). Your care provider will apply the monofilament to each of your feet in five designated areas, as research has shown that people who can sense or feel the monofilament in these locations are at *reduced* risk for developing ulcers. Vibration tests can examine if there is any loss of sensation. All these tests are simple, fast and should be performed on both feet.

In addition, it is extremely important that you perform your own foot and leg examination every day, looking for any changes, discolorations, or breakages in your skin; consider using a mirror so that you can clearly see the bottoms of your feet, and always wear comfortable shoes that fit well.

Sensory nerve damage is painful and, in the extreme, can lead to foot or leg amputation. The best prevention is to maintain good blood glucose control, and be diligent about checking your feet daily, and yearly with your physician.

Treatment of Sensory Neuropathy

The first step in symptom management is to stabilize blood glucose levels. There is evidence that changes in blood glucose may worsen pain, so avoiding swings in your blood glucose levels may help. The next step is to treat the nerve pain. The types of medications that can be used are listed on the next page. Opioid (synthetic narcotic) pain medications are used when the other medications listed in Table 4.4 do not work.

(See next page)

Drug Class	Medication
Pain relievers Over the Counter.	
	aspirin, ibuprofen, naproxen and more
Anticonvulsants Medicines	
	Medicines such as gabapentin
	gabapentin (Gralise)
	gabapentin (Neurontin)
	gabapentin (Horizant)
	pregabalin (lyrica)
	carbamazepine (Tegretol)
Topical Treatments	
	lidocaine cream that is available without a prescription can be applied to the skin.
	capsaici cream
Antidepressants	
	duloxetine (Cymbalta)
	venlafaxine (Effexor XR)
	desvenlafaxine (Pristiq)
	milnacipran (savella)
Narcotic Pain Medications	
	Various pain medication for your physician to pick

Table 4.4 Medications for sensory neuropathy – Not a comprehensive list

What To Know About Your Tests and Exams

Learning about diabetes and its complications is only one part of the educational piece that a person with diabetes needs. The other equally important part is:

- knowing what procedures and lab tests you need

- knowing when they need to be done

- knowing what the results mean, and

- making sure you are prescribed the right medications and making sure you take them.

Diabetic Foot Care

Foot care is very important when you have diabetes. Controlling your blood sugar levels can help you avoid diabetic foot problems. Following some simple guidelines for foot care can make all the difference between healthy feet and amputation. Here are some helpful tips:

1. Check your feet daily. Look for red spots, cuts, swelling, and blisters. Use a mirror or ask for help if you cannot see the bottom of your feet.

2. If sores do not start healing after one day, call your doctor.

3. Wear comfortable, well-fitting shoes and socks. Make sure there is nothing inside them before you put them on.

4. Never walk barefoot.

5. Wash and carefully dry your feet daily.

6. Use lotion to keep the tops and bottoms of your feet soft and smooth. Do not put lotion between your toes.

7. Trim your toenails straight across.

8. Protect your feet from too much hot and cold.

9. Put your feet up when sitting.

10. Do not cross your legs for very long.

11. Wiggle your toes and move your ankles up and down for 5 minutes at least two or three times a day.

ABC MD Foot and Flu

To prevent the complications we have discussed, you need to make sure you do all of your tests, and know your numbers. I have developed a catchphrase or saying to remember these tests and here it is: **ABC MD Foot and Flu.** Say it three or four times to yourself and it will start to stick in your mind. Here is what it stands for:

A	A1C (a minimum of two times a year if controlled; otherwise up to four times a year)
B	Blood pressure (check every time at physician's office and any other opportunity)
C	Cholesterol and creatinine (a minimum once a year)
MD	Medical-Albuminuria (once a year) Dilated eye exam (once a year)
Foot	Foot exam (by your physician once a year)
FLU	Flu shot (once a year)

Now let us look at each of these tests in detail, how to view the results, and your action plan depending on the results.

ABC MD Foot and Flu – A1C

The **A1C** test provides a value for your <u>average blood glucose level</u> over a three-month period of time. ADA guidelines state that this test should be performed at least twice a year. If your A1C is not at goal, then you should test it every three months until you are at goal. The A1C test is done by having your blood drawn at a lab. Your physician must order this test for you. It is different than your daily glucose self-monitoring that you do at home with your glucometer. The A1C test results are related to your home glucose readings. If your home glucose readings are high, your A1C will be high, and vice versa. If you know that these two results (home and lab) are related, then you do not have to wait for an A1C test at the lab to start working on better glucose control. If you start to notice a trend of increasing blood glucose levels, or you are having too many low glucose episodes, it is important to notify your physician so you can work on a plan to control your diabetes.

Another important concept to know about your A1C reading is that you can have an A1C of around 7 percent (generally considered a good reading) and still not really be in control. If you have large glucose swings, for instance, low in the mornings, but high at night, these two readings can counteract each other in your A1C results because the A1C is an average. Let us say you have a morning glucose reading of 58 mg/dl and your nighttime glucose reading is 225 mg/dl. This would give you an average glucose of 141.50 mg/dl, which equates to about 7 percent A1C. But as you can see from the two glucose readings, you are not really in control of your glucose.

Example:

Morning reading: 58 mg/dl
Nighttime reading: 225 mg/dl

    58 + 225 = 283

Divide by 2 to determine the average of the two readings

    283 ÷ 2 = 141.50

A1C Result	Blood Glucose
12	298
11	269
10	240
9	212
8	183
7	154
6	126

Check the A1C chart. 141.50 is roughly equal to 7% A1C (usually considered good control)

But glucose levels of 58 and 225 are _not_ good control!

I am providing you with this example because it is important to make sure your physician is looking at your home glucose readings in conjunction with your A1C results. This is the only way to really see if your A1C reading is the result of stable blood glucose readings, or if it is an average of some really big glucose swings. The glucose swings can be resolved through medication adjustment and diet.

ABC MD Foot and Flu – Blood Pressure

You need to have your **blood pressure** monitored as often as possible. This is because the symptoms of high blood pressure usually cannot be felt and the effects of high blood pressure on the heart, eyes, kidneys, and brain can damage these organs. Every time you visit your physician or have an opportunity to take your blood pressure, you should. The ADA suggests a goal blood pressure for most people with diabetes of less than 130/80 mmHg.

Always ask your physician what your blood pressure is and keep a log of the readings. If it is over 130/80 mmHg, ask for a plan to bring your blood pressure down. If you start with lifestyle changes, such as diet and exercise, and your blood pressure still does not come down to goal, ask your physician about the possibility of using medications to bring it within goal range. It is not unusual for an individual to need more than one medication to bring down blood pressure to goal, so do not be alarmed if this is the case for you. The most important thing to remember is that your blood pressure must be brought to goal because of the damage it may cause to your heart, eyes, kidneys, and brain.

Blood Pressure Ranges

mmHg means millimeters of mercury

Diabetes only	Less than 130/80 mmHg
Diabetes and kidney disease	Possibly less than 125/75 mmHg

ABC MD Foot and Flu – Cholesterol and Creatinine

Cholesterol testing is done by a blood test at the lab that measures several lipid (fat) factors that have an influence on producing disease. This cholesterol testing is sometimes called a lipid panel or lipid profile panel. The results of your lipid panel will include values for: Total cholesterol, HDL, LDL, and triglycerides.

The ADA recommends an annual cholesterol panel. High cholesterol puts you at risk for heart disease and individuals with diabetes are already at higher risk (two to four times) of having heart problems. Also, having high cholesterol does not always produce symptoms that would prompt you to have the test done, so regular testing is very important.

Cholesterol Ranges

Terms: < means less than; > means greater than; mg/dl means milligrams per deciliter; mmol/l means millimoles per liter (an international/scientific unit of measurement)

Total Cholesterol:	Less than 200 mg/dl
HDL:	Males greater than 40 mg/dl \ (1.0 mmol/l)
	Females greater than 50 mg/dl (1.3 mmol/l)
LDL:	No cardiovascular disease = < 100 mg/dl (2.6 mmol/l)
	Has cardiovascular disease = <70 mg/dl (1.8 mmol/l)
Triglycerides level:	Less than 150 mg/dl (1.7 mmol/l)

Ranges for people with diabetes recommended by the American Diabetes Association

A **creatinine** test is a blood test done at the lab to test for kidney function. Serum creatinine should be tested at least once a year in all adults with diabetes, regardless of the degree of urine albumin excretion. Creatinine is a non-protein waste product made by skeletal muscle tissue and is produced continuously in proportion to your muscle mass. It is closely related to the albuminuria test described below. Creatinine is freely filtered by the kidneys; therefore, the serum creatinine level depends on glomerular filtration rate (GFR). When the kidneys are not filtering well, the ability to filter creatinine and excrete it as urine decreases, causing the serum creatinine to rise. Serum creatinine is also used to estimate GFR to determine the level of chronic kidney disease (CKD), if any.

Even though each lab may vary slightly in its acceptable range of values, the ranges listed here are generally accepted.

Serum Creatinine Ranges

Adult males: 0.8 - 1.4 mg/dl.
Males have slightly higher values than females due to larger muscle mass.

Adult females: 0.6 - 1.1 mg/dl.
Females have values lower than males due to smaller muscle mass.

ABC MD Foot and Flu – Medical-albuminuria and Dilated Eye Exam

Make an annual appointment with your doctor for these tests:

Medical-albuminuria

Albuminuria refers to amounts of a protein called

albumin being leaked by the kidneys into the urine. You should be tested yearly for this condition. Albumin in urine indicates the possible beginning of kidney problems and should be taken very seriously to prevent progression albuminuria, in which the kidneys excrete even larger amounts of albumin. Once albuminuria develops, blood pressure will rise slightly and changes to the kidney will likely be irreversible. If no action is taken to decrease or stop the excretion of protein, the kidneys will continue to have a steady decline in the glomerular filtration rate, which leads to end-stage renal disease.

The ADA states that testing for albumin in urine should begin as soon as a person is diagnosed with type 2 diabetes. People with type 1 should be tested every year beginning five years after diagnosis. Screening for albuminuria is performed using a urine test that measures the albumin-to-creatinine ratio in a random spot collection of urine (preferred method); 24-hour or timed collections are more burdensome and add little to prediction of kidney function decline or accuracy of the test.

Ranges for albuminuria

Terms: μg/mg means micrograms per milligram

Normal albuminuria	Less than 30 μg/mg	Normal
Albuminuria	30 – 299 μg/mg	Beginning of damage
Albuminuria	Greater than 300 μg/mg	Damage is certain
Albuminuria	>3,500 ug/g	Severe damage

Dilated Eye Examination

You should have a **dilated eye exam** with a comprehensive eye examination every year. Remember, you need to have this done by an ophthalmologist or an optometrist, not your primary care provider. People with type 2 diabetes should have an initial dilated and comprehensive eye examination shortly after they are diagnosed with diabetes. Individuals with type 1 should have their first dilated and comprehensive eye examination within five years after the onset of diabetes and yearly after that. Diabetic retinopathy is the most frequent cause of new blindness among adults aged 20 to 74 years. Early detection is important to prevent or slow down vision loss before it occurs, and laser photocoagulation surgery can often help.

ABC MD Foot and Flu – Foot Examination

A **foot examination** should be performed at least annually in your physician's office. All adults with diabetes should undergo a comprehensive foot examination to identify high-risk conditions. Your doctor should ask about your history, including any previous foot ulcerations or amputations, nerve or circulation symptoms, impaired vision, tobacco use, and your foot care practices.

Both feet should be examined with your socks and shoes off. Your doctor should start with a general inspection of your skin to see if there are any sores or red pressure points, as well as musculoskeletal deformities. Vascular assessment should include inspection and assessment of foot pulses and testing for loss of protective sensation using the 10-g monofilament plus testing any one of the following: vibration using 128 Hz tuning fork, pinprick sensation, ankle reflexes, or vibration perception threshold.

At home, you should inspect your feet daily. This inspection includes looking at your feet to see if there are any cracks or sores, ingrown toenails, rub marks from your shoes or any unexplained marks on your feet. Being proactive about your self-exams, in conjunction with those performed by your physician will help with early identification of any risk factors for ulcers or amputations.

ABC MD Foot and Flu – Flu Shot

People with diabetes should have a **flu shot** yearly starting at the age of six months, continuing annually unless there are other medical reasons you cannot be given the flu vaccine. Influenza and pneumonia are common, preventable infectious diseases. Any illness you can prevent is a benefit if you have diabetes, especially for those with type 1, since illness affects your blood glucose control.

Since we are talking about vaccinations, this is a good time to discuss the pneumococcal vaccine that helps prevent pneumonia. People with diabetes are at a greater risk to get pneumonia. Ask your physician if this is a vaccine you should receive. Also, you should ask your physician about the covid vaccine and what the latest guidelines say about it. In this fast pace world, guidelines are changing all the time when it comes to infectious diseases ie. Covid. Therefore, ask your physician.

Summary

In many ways, this is one of the most important sections of this book because it outlines in one unit what should be done yearly; ABC MD Foot and Flu. These are the action items that will give you and your physician measurements to be proactive in your diabetes care.

Call your physician today and see if you are current and up to date on all the tests described above. If not, make an appointment for any missing tests to be done and another to go over the results with your physician. At the second visit, you can schedule your six-month follow up visit. See if your physician will give you a lab slip for your second A1C during your current visit, so you can have the test done before you see your physician for your follow up.

It is my sincere hope that you follow the testing schedule that the ADA has developed called, "Standards of Medical Care in Diabetes," which is updated yearly. Without a doubt, knowing your numbers is the key to controlling your diabetes. Your numbers are the only way to know where your strategies are working and where you need to make changes. Note that the tests and testing schedule listed here are the <u>minimum levels</u> of testing for people with diabetes. You may need to perform some of the tests more frequently to make sure you are reaching your goals.

Facts at a glance

1. **Kidneys:** If your kidneys are healthy, there will be no protein or sugar in your urine. Kidney disease in people with diabetes is called diabetic nephropathy.

2. **Eye Damage:** Diabetic retinopathy is the leading cause of blindness among adults between 20 and 74 years of age. Individuals with diabetes are 25 times more likely to become legally blind than individuals who do not have diabetes.

3. **Nerve Damage:** Symptoms such as numbness, tingling or sharp pains in the lower legs or feet may

be signs of nerve damage. Nerve disease in people with diabetes is called diabetic neuropathy. It can lead to amputations in affected areas.

4. **Yearly Tests:** Knowing your numbers is the best way to control your glucose. Following the ABC MD Foot and Flu guidelines on page 136 will help you remember when to get your tests done and how often to do them.

Your Action Plan

Ask your physician to order the following tests to evaluate your kidney function:

- Blood test for creatinine
- Urine test for a protein called albuminuria, or an albumin-to-creatinine ratio and sugar

Ask your physician to give you a thorough foot examination that includes:

- A pinprick sensation test and vibration perception
- Ankle reflex test
- Ankle pulse test

Ask your physician to give you an action plan if a sore or ulcer is discovered on your foot or feet.

Follow the guidelines of ABC MD Foot and Flu (see page 136) and make sure you are getting all of your testing done on time and reviewing the results with your physician.

Chapter 5

Ask Your Physician

It is important to see your physician regularly and be prepared to ask questions about your care. Figure 5.1 listed on the next page is a checklist you can use when you visit your physician, which includes the American Diabetes Association guidelines for each topic. Keep in mind that your targets and goals may be different. Work with your physician to determine what is best for you.

Figure 5.1 Questions for your doctor

Health Topic	Question	Your Notes	ADA RECOMMENDED Goals
A1C Testing	Have you checked my A1C? What is my number and what does it mean? Are we testing enough?		Goal: A1C at 7% or lower[1] If your A1C is 7% or lower, test at least every 6 months. If it is over 7%, test at least every 3 months. If you belong to a special population, your physician may target a different A1C level for you.
Blood Sugar Testing at home	Should I be testing daily? How often and what should the results be?		Blood sugar goal before meals Should be 80-130 mg/dl. Blood sugar goal two hours after meals should be less than 180 mg/dl.
Fasting blood glucose from Lab	What were the last results of my fasting glucose test?		For people without diabetes should be less than 100 mg/dl. A result that is in the range of 100 mg/dl to 126 mg/dl indicates impaired fasting glucose. This indicates you may develop diabetes if you do not get the results under 100 mg/dl. Greater than or equal to 126 mg/dl at two different times indicates diabetes. If you are on medications and your fasting blood glucose is high, you may need to increase the dose or add another medication. Make sure you ask your physician what he is going to do.

References:

1. American Diabetes Association. Clinical Practice Recommendations 2024. Diabetes Care. 2024.

Low blood sugar	What value is considered low blood sugar when I test at home?		A result of less than 70 mg/dl is considered low blood sugar. Treat low blood sugar of 70 mg/dl or less with glucose. Your physician may have a different level for you on what low blood sugar is.
	What are the signs of low blood sugar?		Signs: Tremor, confusion, sweating, headache, difficulty concentrating, rapid heart rate, weakness, and fatigue.
	What do I do if I have low blood sugar?		
	Should you prescribe a glucagon injection kit to recover from low blood sugar?		Your physician should work on a low blood sugar action plan to know exactly what you should do. Once you have this action plan, share it with your family members for help.
			All people who are on insulin should have a glucagon injection kit.
Health Topic	**Question**	**Your Notes**	**ADA RECOMMENDED Goals**
Blood Pressure	Is my blood pressure in the normal range?		The goal for blood pressure is 130/80 mmHg or lower.
	Do I need to take blood pressure medication?		If you are diagnosed with high blood pressure or are not at goal for blood pressure, you should be on medication.
			If you have diabetes and kidney disease with protein in your urine called albuminuria, many experts believe a goal of less than 125/75 may be appropriate.
			If your physician has different blood pressure goals for you, you should know them.

Some blood pressure medications can increase creatinine and potassium in the blood.	Have you tested my blood for serum creatinine and potassium? Is it normal?		This should be checked once a year. If you start a medication for high blood pressure, your serum creatinine and potassium should be rechecked in 3 months. This test also lets the physician know how well the kidneys are working.
Cholesterol	Have you checked my cholesterol?		Goal: LDL cholesterol below 100 mg/dl. Your LDL (bad) cholesterol should be less than 100 mg/dl or less than 70 mg/dl if you have been diagnosed with cardiovascular (heart) disease. Your cholesterol should be checked every year if you are within this range; recheck it in 3 months if your LDL is not within this range. Triglycerides should be less than 150 mg/dl. HDL (good) cholesterol: Men: greater than 40 mg/dl; women: greater than 50 mg/dl.
	Do I need to take medication?		Statin medications are recommended for all patients with diabetes over 40 years of age, and for all patients who have not achieved their LDL goal through lifestyle modifications.
	Once I start a cholesterol medication, how often do you need to test my cholesterol levels?		If you start on a statin medication, you should recheck your cholesterol panel and liver function test after 6 weeks.

Electrolyte panel	Have you checked my electrolytes?		Electrolytes should be done once a year. If you have started on a high blood pressure medication, recheck your electrolyte levels in 3 months. Every time a blood pressure medication is added or there is an increase to your existing medications, wait 3 months and retest.
Eye examination by an optometrist or ophthalmologist	Should I have my eyes checked? How often?		Type 1 diabetes. You should have a complete dilated eye examination initially, then at 5 years of being diagnosed, then every year. Type 2 diabetes. You should have a dilated eye examination soon after being diagnosed. For either type, if your vision is normal, then yearly examinations are recommended. If you have diabetes-related eye problems, your doctor may recommend more frequent examinations.
Kidneys	Have you checked my kidneys? What are the tests?		Urine test for albumin, serum creatinine, and GFR (glomerular filtration rate) are three important tests for kidney function.

Kidney test called Albuminuria	Have you checked my urine for a protein called albuminuria?		Your results should be less than 30 µg/mg and should be checked once a year. If your results are positive for albuminuria, then test every 3-6 months. If any albuminuria is noted, your physician may want to add an ACE inhibitor or an ARB medication even if you do not have high blood pressure.
Thyroid test	Do I need my thyroid levels checked?		If you have type 1 diabetes, you should have your thyroid levels checked. Also, if you feel sad, it is a good idea to have your thyroid checked.
Feet	Should I be checking my feet? How often and what should I do?		Check your feet everyday with your socks and shoes off. Check for loss of feeling, infection, redness, ingrown toe nails and injury. You can use a mirror to check the bottom of your feet for any sores. Have your physician check your feet a minimum of once a year for foot pulse, ankle reflexes and to see if there is any loss of protective sensation.

Weight and Exercise	Should I lose weight? Should I be exercising?		Everyone should check with their physician before starting an exercise program. If you are on insulin or medications that work like insulin, work with your physician on prevention of low blood glucose from exercise. Everyone should have an exercise plan from their physician with types of exercises that are ok to perform and an action plan to follow to prevent or recover from low blood sugars. The ADA recommends that you aim for 150 minutes a week of moderate intense aerobic physical activity (like walking, dancing, or swimming) as tolerated. If you have type 2 diabetes, then you should add a resistance-type exercise (strength training) 3 times a week.
Liver function test (LFT)	Have you checked my liver?		This should be measured when starting a statin medication to lower cholesterol to obtain a baseline reading, and again after 6 weeks of being on the medication. If your results are normal, recheck it once a year.

Health Topic	Question	Notes	ADA Recommended Goals
Vitamin B12 checked	Do I need to check my Vitamin B12?		If you are on Metformin, you should have your vitamin B12 checked annually.
Meal Planning	Should I be following a special diet?		Everyone with diabetes should follow a healthy diet plan. ADA recommends the Diabetes Plate method. ½ of the plate is non-starchy vegetables, ¼ is protein and ¼ is complex carbohydrates. See a dietician for diet, education, and planning.
Feeling "blue" (if applicable)	Lately I have been feeling sad or "down" much of the time. Am I depressed?		Let your physician know if you are feeling sad or "down" much of the time. Your physician will be able to address what medical needs will help you.

A Quick List of Tests and Examinations

Figure 5.2 is a list of tests you might need in order to achieve optimum health and manage your diabetes. Some tests are the minimum required for good control. Other tests will be decided upon by you and your physician, depending on your test results and other factors.

Figure 5.2

TYPE OF TEST	IDEAL RESULTS AND RECOMMENDATIONS
Laboratory Studies	
Blood pressure (BP)	Your goal is less than 130/80 each time you test. If your BP is greater than 130/80, your physician may want to start you on an ACE inhibitor, an ARB, or a combination of medications.
Hemoglobin A1C	This should be less than 7%. If your A1C is less than 7%, recheck it in 6 months. If your A1C is greater than 7%, work with your physician to lower it and recheck it in 3 months.
Fasting blood glucose	For people without diabetes: a goal of less than 100 mg/dl. A result that is in the range of 100 mg/dl to 126 mg/dl indicates impaired fasting glucose. Greater than or equal to 126 mg/dl at two different times indicates diabetes.
Cholesterol (lipid) panel	Your LDL (bad) cholesterol should be less than 100 mg/dl (2.6 mmol/L) (or less than 70 mg/dl [1.8 mmol/L] if you have been diagnosed with cardiovascular disease). Recheck it in 1 year if you are within this range; recheck it in 3 months if your LDL is not within this range. Triglycerides should be less than 150 mg/dl (1.7 mmol/L). HDL (good) cholesterol: Men: greater than 40 mg/dl (1.0 mmol/L); women: greater than 50 mg/dl (1.3 mmol/L). Statin medications are recommended for all diabetic patients over 40 years of age, and for all patients who have not achieved their LDL goal through lifestyle modifications. If you start on a statin medication, you should recheck your cholesterol panel and liver function test after 6 weeks.[2]

Liver function test (LFT)	This should be measured when starting a statin medication to obtain a baseline reading, and again after 6 weeks of being on the medication. If your results are normal, recheck it once a year.
Serum creatinine (SCr)	This should be checked once a year. If you start a medication for high blood pressure, your serum creatinine should be rechecked in 3 months.
Albuminuria test	Your results should be less than 30 µg/mg and should be checked once a year. If your results are positive for albuminuria, then test every 3-6 months. If any albuminuria is noted, your physician may want to add an ACE inhibitor or an ARB medication even if you do not have high blood pressure.
Electrolytes panel	This should be done once a year. If you start on a high blood pressure medication, recheck your electrolyte levels in 3 months.
Vitamin B12	If you are on a medication called Metformin, then you should check your levels of Vitamin B12 yearly.
Foot examination	You should examine your feet yourself every day. A doctor should examine your feet once a year. You can see a podiatrist for this exam or your physician may be able to perform it for you.
Eye examination by an optometrist or ophthalmologist	Type 1 diabetes. You should have a complete eye examination within 3-5 years of being diagnosed. Type 2 diabetes. You should have an eye examination soon after being diagnosed. For either type, if your vision is normal, then yearly examinations are recommended. If you have diabetes-related eye problems, your physician may recommend more frequent examinations.
Psychological examination	It is recommended that you talk to your physician about any problems you may be having in coping with your diagnosis of diabetes and how it affects your life.

Chapter 6

Healthy Eating for People with Diabetes

When you first learned you had diabetes, you may have assumed you would have to go on a special diet and give up all of your favorite foods. In the past, people with diabetes were taught that they could not have any simple carbohydrates, including sugar and fruit, in their diet. Then, in 1994, the American Diabetes Association changed its recommendations to indicate "scientific evidence has shown that the use of sucrose (sugar) as part of the meal plan does not impair blood glucose control in individuals with Type 1 or Type 2 diabetes." This change paved the way to the eating recommendations that are in place today for people with diabetes.

Once you have a better understanding of how food fuels and affects your body, especially your glucose levels, you will see that all foods can fit in your diet. It is the amount (portion) of carbohydrates you eat that significantly affects your blood glucose levels, rather than the type of carbohydrate.

Portion control, as well as carbohydrate control, is important not only to people with diabetes, but to anyone who wants to control their weight. For example, one medium pancake may have 15 grams of carbohydrates and 80 calories compared to one cup of cooked oatmeal, which has 30 grams of carbohydrates and 150 calories. Either food can fit into your meal plan as long as you pay attention to the amount. Practical guidelines to help you with portion control are provided later in this chapter.

In the end, people tend to have better control of their diet and blood sugar when they eat foods they enjoy; the key is to do so in moderation.

The Essentials of Diet

Your body needs an adequate amount of six essential nutrients to function normally. Three of these; water, vitamins and minerals; do not provide any energy and do not affect blood glucose. The other three; carbohydrates, protein, and fat; provide your body with the energy it needs to work and do affect your blood glucose levels. This energy is measured in calories; any food that contains calories will cause your blood sugar to rise. In order for your body to properly use these energy calories it needs insulin. Whenever you eat, your food is digested and broken down into your body's primary fuel source; glucose. While all energy nutrients are broken down into glucose, carbohydrates have a more direct effect on blood glucose levels.

The ADA suggests to simplify healthy eating by using what is called a Diabetes Plate to help with food portions and foods to eat.

A Diabetes Plate is a nine-inch plate and filled half with non-starchy veggies, one-quarter with lean proteins, and one-quarter with quality carbs like starchy vegetables, fruits, whole grains, or low-fat dairy. See example on following page from Diabetes Care 2024.

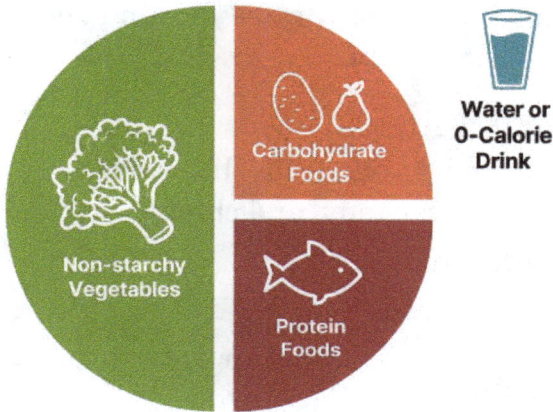

The ADA suggests using the Diabetes Plate as a framework for all the recommended diabetes meal patterns.

Carbohydrates (Carbs)

Carbohydrates are commonly known as starches (complex carbohydrates) and sugars (simple carbohydrates). They are your body's main and preferred source of energy. Carbohydrates enter your bloodstream and give you an immediate energy supply. It is the energy source that affects your blood sugar the most. Foods that contain carbohydrates are grains, fruits and vegetables, dairy foods like milk and yogurt, and sugar.

Complex carbohydrates:

- starchy foods like bread, cereal, rice, and crackers
- starchy vegetables like potatoes and corn
- dried beans like pinto beans, black beans, and lentils

- non-starchy vegetables, which contain small amounts of carbohydrates (but in general are very low)

Simple carbohydrates:

- sweets and snack foods like sodas, juice drinks, cake, cookies, candy, and chips
- fruit and fruit juice
- milk and yogurt

Contrary to popular belief, people with diabetes can have foods with sugar. Carbohydrates are broken down very quickly once you consume them; both sugar and starch end up as glucose. So, you can eat food containing sugar as part of your overall meal plan as long as you account for the carbohydrates and their calories. Of course, foods high in sugar do not have many vitamins and minerals and contain extra calories, which most people do not need.

Sugar-Free Food

People with diabetes often eat "sugar-free" foods thinking they are a healthier alternative to their favorite sweets. These foods replace sucrose (sugar) with sweet tasting substances like sorbitol, mannitol, or xylitol. These are all "sugar alcohols," which are technically not sugar, but are high in carbohydrates. Others may be sweetened with fructose or maltodextrin, which also contain calories and carbohydrates. These foods will affect your blood glucose just as a food containing sugar would. Again, it depends on the total grams of carbohydrates in each serving of the food. In addition, foods containing these sugar alcohols can cause stomach discomfort and diarrhea if eaten in large quantities.

Fiber

Fiber is the indigestible part of plant foods, including fruits, vegetables, whole grains, and legumes. When you consume dietary fiber, most of it passes through the intestines and is not digested. Because it is not broken down by the body, the fiber in an apple or a slice of whole grain bread has no effect on blood glucose levels because it is not digested. Basically, the grams of fiber do not count. If you are counting carbohydrates for meal planning, the grams of fiber can actually be subtracted from the total grams of carbohydrates if you are planning your meals with carb counting. Fiber also delays glucose absorption.

For good health, adults should eat 25 to 30 grams of fiber each day. Most Americans do not consume nearly enough fiber in their diet, eating only about half of the recommended amount. It is best to get your fiber from food rather than taking a supplement. It is important to increase your fiber intake gradually to prevent stomach problems (gas and bloating), and increase your intake of water and other liquids, to prevent constipation. Good sources of dietary fiber include:

- Beans and legumes
- Fruits and vegetables, especially those with edible skin (for example, apples, corn, and beans) and those with edible seeds (for example, berries)
- Whole grains. Because "whole grain" food contains the entire grain kernel; bran, germ, and endosperm; they are much more nutritious than refined grains and have more fiber. "Refined grain" food contains only the endosperm, or the starchy part, so you miss out on many of the vitamins and minerals.

There are two types of fiber:

- Insoluble fiber keeps your digestive tract working well. Whole wheat is an example of this type of fiber.

- Soluble fiber can help lower your cholesterol level and improve blood glucose. Oatmeal and beans are an example of this type of fiber.

Carbohydrate grams

Reading food labels is a great way to know how much carbohydrate is in a food. For foods without a label, you can estimate their carbohydrate content. Keeping general serving sizes in mind will help you estimate how much carbohydrate you are eating. For example, there are about 15 grams of carbohydrate in:

- 1 small piece of fresh fruit (4 oz)
- 1/2 cup of canned or frozen fruit
- 1 slice of bread (1 oz) or 1 (6 inch) tortilla
- 1/2 cup of oatmeal
- 1/3 cup of pasta or rice
- 4 - 6 crackers
- 1/2 English muffin or hamburger bun
- 1/2 cup of black beans or starchy vegetable
- 1/4 of a large baked potato (3 oz)
- 2/3 cup of plain fat free yogurt or sugar free yogurt
- 2 small cookies
- 2-inch square brownie or cake without frosting
- 1/2 cup ice cream or sherbet

- 1 tbsp syrup, jam, jelly, sugar, or honey
- 2 tbsp light syrup
- 1/2 cup soda

As you can see, not all carbohydrate foods are the best choices for you. The preferred sources of carbohydrates are whole grains, vegetables, fruits, and beans because they have the most fiber and give you more nutrients.

Treating Low Blood Sugar

To treat low blood sugar, you need to have carbohydrates that are fast acting and without any fat, so they can be digested immediately and raise your blood sugar quickly. A chocolate candy bar contains fat and takes too long to digest. One 15 gram serving of carbohydrates is needed to treat hypoglycemia. Here are some examples:

- ½ cup juice
- 2 tbsp raisins
- 1 tbsp sugar
- 1 tbsp honey
- 6 Lifesavers
- 1 cup nonfat milk

Glycemic Index (GI)

The glycemic index, or GI, is a system to categorize carbohydrate foods based on how high they raise blood glucose levels after they are eaten. Foods are ranked based on how they compare to a reference food of either glucose or white bread. A food with a high GI raises blood glucose more than a food with a medium or low GI. The GI of a food is different when eaten alone than it is when combined with other food.

- The higher the fiber, the lower the GI of a food.
- Eating a carbohydrate with food that contains fat will cause the carbohydrate to be digested more slowly.
- Fat and protein by themselves do not have carbohydrates and are not ranked on the GI.
- Low-calorie foods, like vegetables, have a small amount of carbohydrates and are not listed on the GI.
- GI can also vary from person to person.

Following are a few examples of other factors that can affect the GI of a food:

1. Ripeness and storage time: The riper a fruit or vegetable is, the higher the GI.
2. Processing: Juice has a higher GI than whole fruit and mashed potatoes have a higher GI than a whole baked potato.
3. Cooking method: How long a food is cooked affects the GI, so al dente pasta has a lower GI than soft-cooked pasta.
4. Type: Short-grain white rice has a higher GI than brown rice.

The GI value represents the type of carbohydrate in a food, but says nothing about the portion of carbohydrate typically eaten. Correct portion sizes are critical in managing blood glucose and losing or maintaining weight. Many nutritious foods have a higher GI than foods with little nutritional value. For example, oatmeal has a higher GI than chocolate. There are many foods with medium or low GIs that are not necessarily the best choices for health, such as ice cream and whole milk. While they are low-GI foods, they are still dense in calories and high in saturated (unhealthy) fat.

Keep in mind that the total amount of carbohydrates you eat and the nutritional value of the food is more important for blood glucose management than their GI. Using the GI may be helpful in "fine-tuning" blood glucose management, just as keeping track of any foods that seem to particularly affect you is a good idea.

To eat a healthy diet and manage your carbohydrate intake you should:

1. Increase intake of fiber and whole grains. Choose 100% whole grain bread and look for fiber content on cereal boxes (3-5 grams or more per serving).

2. Limit eating concentrated sweets, as they have little nutritional value.

3. Eat more fruits and vegetables. The goal is to eat three to four fruits a day and two cups of vegetables per day. Add fruits to breakfast, snacks, and lunch. Add veggies to lunch, snacks, and dinner.

4. Choose healthy beverages. Sugary beverages can really spike your blood sugar and contain extra calories that lead to weight gain. Drink water, unsweetened tea, black coffee, etc. Especially avoid consuming sugary drinks by themselves.

5. Eating carbohydrate foods with foods that contain fat will cause the carbs to be digested more slowly.

As a result, blood glucose will not rise as quickly.

Protein

The second major nutrient your body needs is protein. Protein is primarily used to build and repair your cells and tissues. It is used for energy when there are not enough carbohydrates or fats. However, using protein as an energy source is a long process:

- It takes 3-5 hours after a meal for the protein you have eaten to have any impact on your blood glucose. When carbohydrates and fats are not available for energy usage, or are in short supply, amino acids (the building blocks of protein), can be made into glucose as a back-up energy source.

- It used to be a standard recommendation to have a protein source at every meal and with every snack to slow down the rise of blood glucose. The American Diabetes Association's latest recommendation advises that is not necessary. Again, it is the total amount of carbohydrates eaten at one time that matters.

- Having protein at a meal helps make the meal more nutritious and balanced. It can also help decrease the amount of carbohydrates you need to eat to feel satisfied at mealtimes. For many people, omitting unnecessary protein can help decrease calorie intake and promote weight loss.

Keep your protein intake to only 15-20% of your diet and keep the portions to the size of your fist. Choose proteins that are low in fat:

- Skinless white meat chicken
- Fish

- Turkey breast/ground turkey breast
- Lean beef such as tenderloin or flank steak/London broil
- Lean pork such as center cut pork chops or pork tenderloins
- Beans
- Eggs (especially egg whites)
- Soy foods
- Low-fat dairy (skim or 1% milk, non-fat or low-fat yogurt and cottage cheese)
- Avoid high-fat meats and poultry; trim the fat from meat, take the skin off poultry

High protein diets are still popular, but they are not necessarily healthy. When you eat a large amount of protein, you are consuming less of other food groups and are probably not getting the essential nutrients you need. It usually means you are eating more fat, which can cause a variety of health problems.

The amount of protein in your diet is a concern if you have decreased kidney function or kidney disease. The first sign of kidney disease is spilling small amounts of protein into your urine. If this occurs, you will need to decrease your protein intake.

Fats

The third nutrient your body needs is fat. Fat is used to maintain healthy skin and hair, cushions your organs, carries fat-soluble vitamins through your body, and is a major source of energy when you take in fewer calories than your body needs. Normally, only about 5-10% of the fat you eat is changed into glucose. Fat can affect your blood glucose level in two ways:

1.   Excess fat can increase your body weight. Fat is a concentrated source of calories, so eating too much fat leads to weight gain, which makes you more insulin resistant. When you eat less fat, you can eat a larger quantity of food for the same amount of calories. When eating fat-free versions of foods (such as mayonnaise and salad dressing) check the label to see how many grams of carbohydrates they contain. Keep in mind that these products often have added sugar.

2.   A high-fat meal is digested more slowly than a lower fat meal. This means your blood sugar will rise later after a high-fat meal because the digestion of carbohydrates will be delayed. If you eat a dinner with fried chicken, mashed potatoes and gravy, and biscuits, it may not affect your glucose reading before bedtime. However, during the night, when the high-fat meal finally gets digested, your blood glucose level will rise. This explains why your morning blood sugar reading is high.

The type of fat you choose is important because some fats cause damage to your body and others can be beneficial.

Healthy fats:

- Monounsaturated fats = almonds, olive oil, canola oil, avocado, olives
- Polyunsaturated fats = walnuts, sunflower oil, safflower oil
- Omega-3 fatty acids = fish and fish oil, flaxseed, and flaxseed oil

Unhealthy fats:

- Saturated fats = fatty meats, fried foods, butter, cream, bacon, cheese
- Trans fats (listed as partially hydrogenated oils on ingredient lists) = bakery items, such as cakes, pies, cookies and crackers, chips, fast food, candy, processed and fried foods, and some margarines

Portions and Portion Control

Portions and serving sizes can be very confusing. Determining a healthy portion is easier if you compare it to something you are familiar with such as:

A serving of protein is 3 ounces = the size of a deck of cards or a woman's palm

A serving of fruit = tennis ball or small fist

A serving of raw vegetables is 1 cup = tennis ball or small fist

A serving of starch is ½ cup = golf ball or size of an ice cream scoop

A serving of fat is 1 teaspoon = the size of a penny

A serving of salad dressing is 1 tablespoon = the size of a quarter

Try to keep these visual cues in mind when you are preparing and eating food so that you can moderate your intake of each food group.

How to Read a Food Label

Figure 6.1 shows a typical nutrition label you will find on virtually all food packaging. Make it a healthy habit to read the label when you are choosing what to buy and look for this information when you dine out as well. More and more restaurants are making this information available on their menus or at your table so you can make better decisions about what you order.

You will want to look for foods that are higher in fiber, protein, and vitamins, and lower in calories, fat, and cholesterol.

Here is a sample food label.

Nutrition Facts

Serving Size 1 cup (228g)
Servings Per Container 2

Amount Per Serving

	% Daily Value
Total Fat 12g	18%
Saturated Fat 3g	15%
Trans Fat 3g	
Cholesterol	
Sodium 470mg	20%
Total Carbohydrate 31g	10%
Dietary Fiber 1g	4%
Sugars 5g	
Protein 7g	
Vitamin A	4%
Vitamin C	2%
Calcium	20%
Iron	4%

Serving Size
This tells you the size of 1 serving, not the whole package. Learn to "see" what a serving size looks like, for example:

This amount of food...	is about the size of...
1 cup whole grain cereal	a fist
3 ounces of meat	a deck of cards
1 cup of whole wheat pasta	a tennis ball
½ cup cooked brown rice	a baseball

Servings per Container
- This tells you how many servings are in the package
- *Be careful* – most packages have more than 1 serving

Check Calories
This tells you how many calories are in one serving, not the whole package. There are 2 servings in this example. Total calories are 190.

Limit These Nutrients to Help Protect Your Heart
Total Fat, Cholesterol, and Sodium

Get Enough of These Nutrients for Better Health
Dietary Fiber, Vitamin A, Vitamin C, Calcium, and Iron

Talk with your physician or dietitian about your food plan. Working together will help you create a plan that you can follow every day.

Almost all packaged foods have a food label called Nutrition Facts. Knowing how to read these labels can help you:

- Make healthier food choices
- Know how much you can eat
- Control your weight

Weight Loss

Studies show that losing even a modest amount of weight (just 5-10% of your body weight) can help prevent the progression from pre-diabetes to type 2 diabetes. For a 200-pound person, that means a weight loss of just 10 to 20 pounds could be the difference between developing diabetes or not. Your body is better able to respond to insulin and get glucose out of the blood and into your cells if you lose weight.

Exercise

Exercise is great for people with diabetes and should be part of your treatment plan. It improves your blood sugar, reduces insulin resistance, and can promote weight loss.

When you are active your muscles are working harder and need more energy. During the first ten minutes of exercise, most of your energy needs come from glucose stored in your muscles, which is called glycogen. As you continue to exercise there is less glycogen available, so your body begins to use glucose from your blood and fat from your fat stores. This process helps you continue exercising. Thirty minutes of activity generally lowers your blood glucose by about 30 mg/dl. After you finish exercising, your muscles replace glycogen stores for up to 24 hours. You may get low blood sugar from exercise and may need to eat extra carbohydrates.

- If you are on insulin or take a sulfonylurea medication that helps your pancreas produce more insulin (glyburide, glipizide, or glimepiride), you may need to eat more carbohydrates before, during or after exercise to avoid getting hypoglycemia.

- Check your blood glucose before you exercise. If it is below 100, you will want to have a snack that contains some carbohydrates. You may also need to adjust your medication or insulin to avoid dropping too low. Talk to your physician about a plan that is right for you.

- To help prevent low blood glucose, check it about every 30 to 45 minutes after exercise to gauge whether your blood glucose is going down, going up, or leveling off. If it is going down, eat a small serving of carbohydrates and keep checking until you level off. You may experience low blood sugar up to 24 hours after exercise.

- It is common to need less diabetes medication as you exercise and lose weight. Monitor your blood sugar and let your doctor know if your blood sugar is getting too low.

- If you do not take a sulfonylurea or insulin, you most likely will not have hypoglycemia while exercising. Having extra carbohydrates may not be needed, and may slow down any weight loss benefits from exercise.

Recommendations:

- Set small goals so that you can find activities you like to do.

- Make time in your day for physical activity.
- Gradually work up to exercising at least five times a week for 30 to 45 minutes per day.
- Examples of physical activity include: walking, dancing, gardening, hiking, group exercise classes (step, kickboxing, Zumba, yoga, water aerobics, etc.)

The number one requirement is that you find something which you really enjoy doing so that you can stick with it. Doing several different activities throughout the week may help you avoid becoming bored with your exercise program.

Summary

Balanced meals (with whole grains, proteins, and healthy fats) are harder for your body to break down. Therefore, glucose from carbohydrates will be absorbed into the bloodstream more slowly and over a longer period of time. Instead of a high spike, you get a slower rise in blood sugar, and you will not experience the sharp drop in blood glucose associated with foods high in sugar. Slow absorption of glucose provides continual energy over several hours, leading to less frequent hunger, more sustained blood sugars, and fewer cravings for high sugar or high fat foods. A balanced diet results in fewer cravings, less hunger, less insulin spikes and less fat storage.

Tips on Eating Right

- Eat at about the same time every day. Regular mealtimes help keep your insulin or medicine and sugar levels steady.

- Try to eat three times a day. Avoid snacks unless you are exercising or treating hypoglycemia.
- If you are overweight, lose weight. Even losing just a little weight, such as 5 to 15 pounds, can lower your blood sugar levels.
- Eat plenty of fiber. Green leafy vegetables, whole grains and fruits are good choices. Fiber helps you feel full and aids digestion.
- Eat fewer empty calories, such as alcohol, and foods high in sugar and fat.

Healthy eating with diabetes requires some work, and it is normal to feel overwhelmed at first. Do not try to do it all right away; instead, make one change at a time, and focus on what you can do to keep going in the right direction. Keep in mind that changing your diet is often a trial-and-error process; eventually, you will find what works for you. Your resolve to live a healthier life through good eating habits will reward you for years to come.

Chapter 7

Medications

Introduction

A well-rounded diabetes educational program gives you the knowledge to understand diabetes, to know what happens when you do and do not have control of your disease, and provides the tools to be in command of your diabetes management. The final piece of this program is a review of the medications that are so necessary for good diabetes management. This chapter aims to bridge the gap between understanding diabetes and achieving diabetes control through the correct use of these medications.

I have noticed that many people do not like to take medication, because they believe it means their health is worsening or that somehow, they have been "bad." They see medication as a punishment or penalty for not doing better with their disease. Or they may believe that functioning with little or no medication must be "better," and that this is somehow a symbol of being healthier. While this attitude might seem logical on the surface, I believe that the opposite is actually closer to the truth.

If you agree with me that your prime directive is to bring your diabetes under control, then medication becomes your ally, not your foe. When an individual has a chronic disease like diabetes, lifestyle changes, such as diet and exercise, just may not be enough to gain control. This does not mean you have been "bad" or have somehow failed, and it does not necessarily mean your condition is worsening. It simply means that diabetes is a strong opponent and you will need to go even further to win the battle. In this light, medications are an integral tool to bring diabetes under control and prevent complications.

There is no doubt that hyperglycemia causes complications for people with diabetes. The relationship between high blood glucose levels and chronic microvascular disease, such as retinopathy (eye), nephropathy (kidney), and neuropathy (nerves) has been demonstrated in large clinical studies. Beyond this, the statistics indicate that individuals with diabetes have a two to four times increase in cardiovascular complications as well. So, if medications can control diabetes and prevent or slow the progression of complications, then there is no reason to avoid them; in fact, they can help you achieve your diabetes goals more quickly.

One of the most important factors in adopting medication as part of your regime is to realize that sometimes as many as three or four medications are necessary to control the various mechanisms that play a role in diabetes. If that is the case for you, do not worry. Your goal is to bring your diabetes under control so that you can stay healthy and live your life to the fullest. It also means that if insulin is the only medication that will decrease your A1C enough to get in control, then it is the right medication for you.

Today there are many different medications you can use to decrease blood glucose levels and raise insulin sensitivity. Each medication has a unique way of working in your body, called a mechanism of action (MOA). Because of the different mechanisms of action, your physician will work with you to determine the right medication or medications for you. He or she may look at patterns in your blood glucose levels, how high your levels are, how long you have had diabetes and how well you might tolerate each medication. Your knowledge of different medications will help you to understand why your physician has chosen a certain drug for you, and also empowers you to ask about other drugs and their ability to get you to your goal. I will not go over every drug available, but most of the major drug classes will be reviewed. With all of this in mind, I want to emphasize that the information provided in this chapter is meant to enhance your knowledge of diabetes medications for hyperglycemia and is not intended to replace your physician's advice.

Fasting Vs. Postprandial Hyperglycemia

Postprandial levels refer to readings taken after eating. Fasting glucose levels refer to readings taken after approximately eight hours without food or drink (except water). When determining which medication to prescribe for your diabetes, your physician will probably first want to evaluate your fasting and postprandial glucose levels. Fasting and postprandial hyperglycemia require different types of medications to bring down blood glucose, so these two types of readings are important factors in determining what medication is best for you.

If you have high blood glucose when you are fasting, it indicates that glucose is being produced mostly by your liver and, to a lesser degree, by your kidneys. Fasting hyperglycemia occurs when there is more glucose in the bloodstream than the body can use. In people without diabetes, glucose levels decrease when they are fasting or not eating. As blood glucose decreases, insulin levels decrease proportionately. This makes sense, because there is no need for large amounts of insulin when no food is present.

The decrease in insulin signals your body to find another way to get the energy it needs, which results in two major actions by the body:

1. An increase in adipose (fat) and muscle tissue breakdown to provide products that can be used to make glucose in the liver; and

2. A decrease in the ability of cells to use glucose, making more glucose available for the brain.

This is an important mechanism to protect the brain, since glucose is its main energy source. This delicate balance is not maintained in individuals with diabetes because the amount of insulin secreted relative to the amount of glucose present is not effective. This may be caused by insulin resistance or an inability to secrete insulin.

Your brain is further protected because it is not dependent on insulin to utilize glucose the way other cells are. The brain is non-insulin-dependent. In individuals without diabetes, the plasma insulin level stabilizes at a level in which glucose production equals the brain's need for glucose. In other words, the amount of insulin produced will not exceed a level that will decrease glucose production below what the brain needs to function. Blood glucose levels are determined by the rate of glucose production from the liver and kidney because the rate of glucose utilization by the brain is fixed.

Postprandial glucose levels occur after you eat. High glucose levels from food increase insulin secretion to allow the absorption of glucose into the cells. A high postprandial glucose level indicates that more insulin is required for glucose to be utilized by the body from the food being eaten. This insulin requirement is much larger than in the fasting state.

In individuals who have had type 2 diabetes for years, insulin is not working as effectively as it should due to insulin resistance. The pancreas starts to increase the secretion of insulin to compensate for the high blood glucose. As the pancreatic beta cells work harder and harder to put out more insulin, they start to burn out. The remaining cells must secrete more insulin to make up the difference. Eventually, the remaining cells are also destroyed. The deterioration of the beta cells not only affects insulin secretion after meals, but will affect insulin secretion throughout the day, which is called basal insulin secretion. After a number of years, if blood glucose is not controlled, individuals will become severely insulin deficient due to beta cell destruction and will require insulin replacement therapy.

The goal of any medication is to bring the body back as close as possible to its normal healthy function. With diabetes, the goal is to mimic the body's natural response to glucose to gain good glucose control. A high postprandial glucose level, whether in type 1 or type 2, indicates that medication should be directed to handle high glucose at that time. If you have high glucose when you are not eating, (sleeping, fasting for eight or more hours, or in between meals), this means your liver is producing excess glucose. Therefore, medications that slow down the liver's glucose production should be chosen.

General Medication Information

Before taking any medication, you should examine the basic information about it, such as contraindications and warnings, side effects or adverse reactions, drug interactions, mechanism of action, route of administration, and danger black box warning. This information should be included when you get your prescription filled at a pharmacy. If not, ask your pharmacist to provide it. Here is what these terms mean:

Contraindication: Advises when a medication is known to cause harm and, not indicated (advised) for a patient who has certain diseases, conditions, or allergies.

Warning: States that a drug or chemical has the potential to cause harm and should be used with caution.

Side Effect or Adverse Reaction: A possible reaction has been noticed in individuals taking the medication, which can range from being mild (like nausea) to very severe.

Drug Interaction: When two drugs used together cause or change the way either medication works or side effects, the result can be either desirable or undesirable.

Mechanism of Action: The way the drug works in the body; the pathway it takes to achieve the intended results.

Route of Administration: How you take the medicine, for example, orally (by mouth), topical (on your skin), or subcutaneous injection (a shot).

Black Box Warning: This information tells you if there are medical studies that indicate whether the drug carries a significant risk of serious or even life-threatening adverse effects. If the medication is still on the market, then these serious effects are usually rare, but the Food and Drug Administration (FDA) feels you have a right to know of the potential danger.

Classes of Diabetes Medications

All medications prescribed by physicians are grouped into drug classes. Each drug class is specific by the way the drug works in the body. If you know the name of the drug class, then you know how the drug works. The diabetic medications listed here are grouped into five main classes. They are:

1. **Biguanide** - Lowers the liver's production of glucose and increases insulin sensitivity in peripheral tissues. It is administered orally (by mouth).

2. **Sulfonylurea/Meglitinide** - Increases insulin secretion from the pancreas. It is administered orally.

3. **Thiazolidinedione** - Enhances insulin sensitivity at muscle, liver, and fat cells, and suppresses glucose production in the liver. It is administered orally.

4. **Insulin** - Provides insulin. It is administered by subcutaneous injection (a shot).

5. **Amylin, GPL-1, and DPP-4 inhibitors** – Increase other hormones in the body that affect glucose levels. GLP-1 and amylin-type medications are

administered by injection and DPP-4 inhibitors are given orally.

6. **SGLT2 inhibitors** – Cause the kidney to pee out glucose, thus reducing glucose in the blood stream.

The key is to understand how these medications work and how effective they are at lowering your A1C so that you can talk to your physician about whether they will get you to goal. The closer you get to goal, the less likely you are to develop complications.

Remember, your mission is to bring your glucose down to the A1C goal your physician determines for you, or the American Diabetes Association (ADA) goal of less than 7%. As each medication class is reviewed, it is important that you pay special attention to how much your A1C will be lowered by the drug, and if it is enough to reach your goal. For example:

- If a drug has the potential to decrease A1C from 0.5% to 1.0%, this means that it will decrease your A1C level by 0.5 to 1.0 points.

- So, if your A1C is at 9.5%, the potential reduction would bring your A1C to 8.5% to 9.0%.

Did that get you to goal? Not if your goal is 7%. Therefore, you will need another medication to bring down the A1C. The ADA recommends insulin if the A1C is > 10% or blood glucose $\geq$ 300 mg/dl, and the person's symptoms of high glucose are detrimental. Of all the medications listed, insulin is the only one that has no limitation on how much it can bring down A1C.

As you look over this list and when you discuss medications with your physician, please remember to ask these five questions:

- What is the name of the drug?
- How does the drug work?
- How much can it lower my A1C?
- What are the side effects?
- Does the drug get me to goal?

1. Class of Medication: Biguanide

Common Names:

Brand Name	Generic Name
Glucophage	metformin

How it Works: Metformin decreases liver glucose production, reduces insulin resistance, decreases mainly fasting hyperglycemia in type 2 diabetes, does not cause weight gain and often improves lipid profile.

A1C Reduction: It reduces A1C approximately 1.5%. This medication is primarily for individuals with type 2, although few physicians have prescribed it to individuals with type 1 to increase insulin sensitivity.

Comments: The American Diabetes Association ranks metformin as the first drug of choice to treat type 2 diabetes. This means that the American Diabetes Association has created guidelines for doctors indicating that metformin should be prescribed first, unless the patient has other issues that indicate it should not be used.

Side Effects: The side effects associated with metformin are gastrointestinal symptoms, most commonly a metallic taste, loss of appetite, nausea, and diarrhea. These symptoms will decrease over time; starting at a low dose will help to lessen symptoms.

Route of Administration: Orally (by mouth).

Contraindications/Caution: Individuals with impaired renal function with a serum creatinine equal to or greater than 1.5 in men, or equal to or greater than 1.4 in women cannot use this medication. A decreased oxygen state, such as heart failure or severe respiratory insufficiency, and severe liver disease may be contraindicated. Caution in elderly.

Black Box Warning: There is a rare possibility of lactic **acidosis** usually related to decreased kidney function.

2. Class of Medication: Insulin Secretagogues: Sulfonylureas/Meglitinides

Common Names:

Brand Name	Generic Name
Sulfonylureas	the three Gs
Amaryl	glimepiride
Glucotrol	glipizide
Micronase, Glynase, DiaBeta	glyburide
Meglitinides	
Prandin	repaglinide
Starlix	nateglinide

Sulfonylureas and Meglitinides

How it Works: There are two groups of medications that increase insulin secretion called insulin secretagogues: sulfonylureas and meglitinides. They help reduce blood glucose levels by increasing insulin secretion. Insulin secretagogues stimulate the beta cells of the pancreas to increase insulin secretion. The major factors to consider between the two groups is how fast the medication works, how long it works, and adverse reactions. This type of medication can only be given to individuals with type 2 diabetes. It does not work in type 1 diabetes because the beta cells on the pancreas do not work.

A1C Reduction: The sulfonylureas reduce A1C by 1.0% to 1.5%, while the meglitinides reduce A1C by 0.6% to 0.7%.

Comments: Do not skip meals when taking these drugs because of the increased risk of low blood sugar. The sulfonylurea group is more commonly used than meglitinides, but if you are allergic to sulfa drugs you cannot use the sulfonylureas (glipizide, glyburide or glimepiride). Glipizide is safest for those with poor kidney function. The meglitinides (Prandin and Starlix) have a faster onset and shorter duration of activity.

Side Effects: Hypoglycemia due to the increase in insulin secretion.

Route of Administration: Orally (by mouth).

Contraindications/Caution: Frequent hypoglycemia, type 1 diabetes, and diabetic ketoacidosis. Sulfonylureas cannot be used if one has an allergy to sulfa drugs. Caution in renal and liver impairment.

Black Box Warning: None

3. Class of Medication: Thiazolidinedione (TZD)
Common Names:

Brand Name	Generic Name
Actos	pioglitazone

How it Works: Thiazolidinedione (commonly referred to as TZD) decreases insulin resistance in the body and around the liver resulting in decreased liver glucose output in the presence of insulin. Secondary benefits are a reduction in plasma free fatty acids, a decrease in liver triglyceride content, and improvement in lipid profile. They are prescribed to individuals with type 2 diabetes.

A1C Reduction: The A1C reduction for pioglitazone is 0.9% to 1.9%. For rosiglitazone it is 0.8% to 1.5%.

Comments: People on insulin and TZD have a greater potential for edema (fluid retention) than TZDs alone. Monitor weight gain and talk to your physician if you have unexplained weight gain and/or edema.

Side Effects: The major side effect is fluid retention with peripheral edema and, in unusual circumstances, congestive heart failure and weight gain. Mild to moderate peripheral edema is observed in 3% to 5% of patients treated with TZD alone. This increases to approximately 15% in patients treated with a combination of pioglitazone and insulin.

Route of Administration: Orally (by mouth).

Contraindications/Cautions: Individuals with symptomatic congestive heart failure (CHF) and CHF class III – IV should not be on TZDs. Caution in individuals with liver impairment, edema, or on insulin.

Black Box Warning: Both drugs have a black box warning that they can cause or increase congestive heart failure; rosiglitazone has an additional black box warning for possible risk of heart attack or increased angina.

4. Class of Medication: Insulin

There are four different groups of insulins, which are characterized by how quickly and how long they work. They are:

1. Rapid-acting

2. Short-acting

3. Intermediate-acting

4. Long-acting

The different time-action profiles of insulin make it possible to pursue the goal of simulating insulin secretion as seen in people without diabetes. Insulin therapy should be thought of in terms of mealtime (bolus) and basal (24 hour a day) insulin therapy.

Mealtime:

Rapid-acting or short-acting human insulins are used for mealtime dosing. They are used in an attempt to simulate the high levels of insulin seen in individuals without diabetes after eating.

Basal:

Intermediate and long-acting human insulins are used for basal insulin therapy to provide a long duration of action and coverage throughout the day. They simulate the basal level of insulin (a baseline level of insulin throughout the day) seen in individuals without diabetes when they are not eating (between meals, through the night and fasting).

Approximate Effects of Insulin:

Not a comprehensive list

Brand Name	Generic Name	Onset of Action	Peak Effect	Duration of Action
Rapid-acting				
NovoLog	Insulin aspart	10-30 min	30-90 min	3.5 hrs
Humalog	Insulin lispro	10-30 min	30-90 min	3-5 hrs
Apidra	Insulin glulisine	10-30 min	30-90 min	3-5 hrs
Fiasp	Insulin aspart	15 min	60-90 min	5-6 hrs
Tresiba	Insulin inhaled	12 min	35-45 min	1.5-3 hrs
Short-acting				
Humulin R	Insulin Regular	30-60 min	1.5-2 hrs	5-8 hrs
Novolin R	Insulin regular	30-60 min	1.5-2 hrs	5-8 hrs

Intermediate-acting (NPH)				
Humulin N	Insulin NPH	1-2 hrs	4-8 hrs	10-20 hrs
Novolin N	Insulin NPH	1-2 hrs	4-8 hrs	10-20 hrs
Long-acting				
Levemir	Insulin detemir	1 hr	Relatively flat peak	12-20 hrs
Lantus	Insulin glargine	1-2 hrs	No peak	22-24 hrs
Tresiba	Insulin degludec	1-2 hrs	No Peak	Up to 42hr

Rapid-Acting, Short-Acting, Intermediate-Acting

How it Works: Stimulates peripheral glucose uptake, inhibits liver glucose production, inhibits the breakdown of adipose tissue, and regulates glucose metabolism.

A1C Reduction: There is no limit to how much insulin can lower your A1C. Therefore, insulin has the greatest ability to decrease A1C.

Comments: Intermediate-acting or long-acting insulin is used for regulating basal (24-hour) insulin coverage. Long-acting insulin is preferred. It allows the individual to give one injection per day, usually at night, for all day basal coverage. This regimen is convenient and easy and has been added to many type 2 diabetes treatment plans in addition to the oral medication. Meal-related insulin secretion stimulates glucose utilization and storage, which decreases glucose production from the liver. Rapid- and short-acting insulins are used for regulating mealtime glucose levels. Insulin can be given to people with type 1 or type 2 diabetes.

Side Effects: Hypoglycemia.

Route of Administration: Subcutaneous injection (a shot).

Contraindications: Hypoglycemia.

Black Box Warnings: None

5. **Class of Medication: Incretin class which consist of three groups of medications: GLP-1, DPP4 inhibitors, and Amylin**

This group consists of three types of medications: GLP-1, DPP-4 inhibitors, and Amylin. They are among the newest drugs in diabetes control. A number of enzymes and hormones were found to be involved in the metabolism when food is ingested and absorbed in the gastrointestinal tract. Some of these hormones are produced in the GI tract and are called incretins, which regulate normal body functions affecting glucose levels. Amylin is another hormone that is produced from beta cells which also is produced by food intake.

How it Works: The mechanism of action of incretins is to stimulate insulin secretion, suppress glucagon secretion (leads to decrease glucose output by the liver), inhibit gastric emptying (slows food leaving the stomach), and reduce appetite and food intake. These drugs only work in the presence of glucose from food and, therefore, are said to be glucose dependent. This medication is used in individuals with type 2 diabetes.

Incretin: GLP-1

Today we have medications that mimic the GLP-1 hormone. The limitation with GLP-1 produced by the body is that its effect is very short, because it is quickly broken down by an enzyme called dipeptidyl peptidase-4 (DPP-4). The drugs below perform the same way as GLP-1 produced in the body, but have been modified to last longer.

GLP-1 Names:

Brand Name	Generic Name
Byetta	exenatide
Victoza	liraglutide
Bydureon	exenatide
Trulicity	dulaglutide
Ozempic	semaglutide

A1C Reduction: GLP-1 reduces A1C by 0.5% to 1.1%.

Comments: These drugs enhance insulin secretion and glucagon suppression in the presence of food that provides glucose to the intestine and, therefore, are glucose dependent. This means that as glucose concentrations fall back to normal ranges, the drug's effect on insulin secretion and glucagon suppression (decreased liver glucose) is diminished.

Side Effects: Nausea, vomiting, constipation, stomach upset, headache, and GERD (gastroesophageal reflux disease).

Route of administration: These drugs are given by subcutaneous injection (shot) and are only for individuals with type 2 diabetes.

Contraindications/Caution: These drugs are contra-indicated in type 1 diabetes, and for those with diabetic ketoacidosis, gastroparesis, a history of pancreatitis, or severe renal impairment.

Black Box Warning: There is a black box warning of thyroid C cell tumor risk.

Incretin: DPP-4 Inhibitor

The DPP-4 inhibitor drugs block the enzyme that breaks down the body's own incretin hormones (GLP-1 and GIP), thereby increasing insulin release and a decrease in glucagon levels. Suppression of glucagon leads to decrease glucose output by the liver. It also slows food leaving the stomach, which reduces appetite and food intake. These medications are used in individuals with type 2 diabetes.

Common Names:

Brand Name	Generic Name
Januvia	sitagliptin
Onglyza	saxagliptin
Nesina	alogliptin
Tradjenta	linagliptin

A1C Reduction: The decrease in the A1C for sitagliptin is 0.6% to 0.8% and for saxagliptin is 0.3% to 0.9%.

Comments: These medications enhance the duration of effectiveness of your body's own GLP-1 and GIP hormones. These hormones are activated when glucose enters the intestines such as after a meal, thus it is glucose dependent. They stimulate insulin secretion, suppress glucagon secretion, slow gastric emptying, and reduce appetite and food intake. There is not a large A1C drop with these drugs, but they have no effect on weight.

Side Effects: Gastrointestinal upset, but less than Byetta or Victoza.

Route of Administration: These medications are taken orally.

Contraindications/Cautions: Contraindicated in type 1 diabetes, and diabetic ketoacidosis. Caution in renal impairment and if there is a history of pancreatitis.

Black Box Warnings: There are no black box warnings.

Amylin

Amylin is a hormone that is released by the beta cells of the pancreas and contributes to glucose control at mealtime. Symlin is a drug that mimics amylin's action in the body. This drug is only used in individuals who use insulin at meal time to control their glucose. Therefore, it can be used in type 1 or type 2 diabetes. It slows gastric emptying (food leaving your stomach), prevents postprandial rise in glucagon, and helps decrease food intake by signaling the brain that you are full.

Common Names:

Brand Name	Generic Name
Symlin	pramlintide

A1C Reduction: Symlin can reduce A1C by 0.5%-0.6%.

Comments: In people with type 1 diabetes, Symlin is used in patients who also use mealtime insulin, but who do not yet have good glucose control. In people with type 2 diabetes, it is also used for those patients who take mealtime insulin but do not achieve good control with or without metformin or sulfonylureas.

Side Effects: Gastrointestinal upset (nausea, vomiting) and headache.

Route of Administration: The drug is given by subcutaneous injection (a shot).

Contraindications: A confirmed diagnosis of gastroparesis (a reduced ability of the stomach to empty) or hypoglycemia.

Black Box Warning: Severe hypoglycemia when used with insulin.

6. Class of Medication: Sodium-glucose cotransporter 2 (SGLT2) called SGLT2 Inhibitor

SGLT2 Inhibitors
Common names

Brand Name	Generic Name
Invokana	canagliflozin
Jardiance	empagliflozin
Steglatro	ertugliflozin
Farxiga	dapagliflozin

A1C Reduction: The decrease in the A1C is 0.5% to 0.7%.

Comments: Sodium-glucose cotransporter 2 (SGLT2), expressed in the proximal renal tubules, is responsible for the majority of the kidney to reabsorb filtered glucose from the tubular that concentrates urine. By inhibiting SGLT2, these medications reduce reabsorption of glucose and thereby promotes glucose to be eliminated through the urine.

Side Effects: Urinary tract infections, and GI symptoms

Route of Administration: These medications are taken orally.

Contraindications/Cautions: Contraindicated in type 1 diabetes, and diabetic ketoacidosis. Caution in renal impairment and if there is a history of pancreatitis.

Black Box Warnings: There are no black box warnings.

Summary

The purpose of any of the medications we have discussed is to decrease blood glucose. The most important question is this: Are the medications you are presently taking getting you to goal? If not, you need to reevaluate whether your medications have enough A1C reduction capability to get you where you need to go. Also, make sure that you are taking all of your medications properly and at the right time every day.

It is important to know that most medications that decrease A1C do not have the ability to decrease the A1C more than 1.5% by themselves. Also, taking a medication that lowers your A1C by one point and another drug that lowers it by one point does not always mean you will see a two-point reduction. In other words, the effects of the drugs are not always cumulative. Therefore, it is very important to be consistent with blood glucose testing to see the results of new or added medications. If you have an A1C of 10 or greater, it is very important you consult a physician and/or endocrinologist.

Remember, along with diet and exercise, your medications are your ally in your efforts to control your diabetes. They are a great tool to bring your glucose, and thus your A1C, into a healthy range so you can prevent complications.

Chapter 8

Insulin

Introduction

I may be biased, but I think the discovery of insulin was one of the greatest breakthroughs of modern medicine. What is particularly amazing is that it occurred only a short time ago. In 1921, four Canadian researchers at the University of Toronto discovered insulin as a treatment for diabetes. The first human injection was given the following year. Then, in 1936, another advance took place when Danish researcher Hans Christian Hagedorn discovered that placing insulin in a mixture (fish protamine suspension) allowed it to be absorbed more slowly in the body, resulting in a longer lasting effect. Following this, in 1946, Canadians D.A. Scott and A.M. Fisher added zinc to the protamine mixture, extending the absorption time even further, leading to the development of NPH (neutral protamine Hagedorn) insulin, which is still used today.

For the next 60 years, insulin was available only in cow (bovine) or pig (porcine) preparations, which closely resembled actual human insulin. In 1980, however, an exact match for human insulin was synthesized using recombinant DNA. In the 1990s, insulin products with faster action were produced to more closely mimic the physiologic (normal body) action of insulin after eating. Lispro, the first rapid-acting insulin approved by the FDA, was developed in 1996, followed by Aspart in 2000 and Apidra in 2004. The availability of rapid-acting insulin allowed for mealtime insulin treatment, which provides better glucose control after a meal. At the same time, long-acting insulin was developed: Lantus in 2000 and Levemir in 2005. These two insulins provided coverage throughout the day during non-meal times.

When you think about this timeline, you can see that the treatment of diabetes is relatively new; prior to 1922, there was no treatment for this disease; people simply died from it. Researchers today continue to study the intricate relationships of insulin in the body with the hope of developing even better delivery systems for this pivotal element of diabetes treatment.

Administering Insulin

The discovery of rapid- and long-acting insulin medication provided the first means of delivering insulin in a form that closely mimics the action of insulin produced in people without diabetes. You can imagine how this provides better treatment for individuals with type 1 diabetes since the drug list for lowering glucose in type 1 diabetes is very short: Insulin. However, not everyone with diabetes is on an insulin regimen. Using insulin requires that you be self-motivated, willing to monitor your glucose several times a day, as well as making sure you understand insulin dosing. There are several schedules that can be used for an insulin dosing regimen, but here we will only discuss prandial or bolus (mealtime) and basal (the low rate of insulin required throughout the day to perform basic metabolic functions) insulin treatment plans.

As you have already learned, in people without diabetes insulin is continuously secreted by the pancreas throughout the day, but two distinct patterns emerge: one at mealtime, and one at other times of the day. At mealtime, the body senses glucose within ten minutes of eating and starts to secrete a little bit of insulin. As the meal progresses and more glucose is present, the pancreas provides a larger amount of insulin to accommodate the intake of food.

At non-mealtimes, such as during sleep, the pancreas secretes a small continuous amount of insulin (the basal rate) to control the glucose being produced by the liver. This pattern of insulin coverage is what you and your physician will try to mimic with your insulin dosing, especially in people with type 1 diabetes where both basal and prandial (meal-related) insulin secretion is absent.

Insulin is always given by injection because your stomach acid would destroy the insulin if it were in pill form. Each type of insulin has a different potency or strength, which is measured in units. In the United States and many other countries, the preparation of insulin contains 100 units per milliliter (units/ml) and is known as U-100 insulin. Most insulin vials prescribed are in small bottles of 10 ml. For people who need large doses of insulin, there are highly concentrated U-500 insulin (500 units/ml) vials. Different insulins also act in different ways in the body. This is known as the profile of action. These profiles reflect how quickly and how long the insulin is effective in your body.

The Four Classifications of Insulin

Insulin medications fall into four classifications, categorized by how fast they work.

- Rapid-acting
- Short-acting
- Intermediate-acting
- Long-acting

Within each of these classifications there are three main criteria that affect the absorption of insulin, which are:

- Onset of action – the length of time it takes for the insulin to start to work
- Peak action – the length of time the insulin is most effective
- Duration of action – the length of time the insulin still has some effect in your body

Mealtime or prandial insulin, often called bolus insulin, can either be rapid-acting insulin (Aspart, Lispro or Apidra) or short-acting insulin (Humulin R or Novolin R). As the name implies, rapid-acting insulin has the fastest onset of action, the fastest peak and the shortest duration. These traits are important because when you eat a meal, your goals are to:

a. control the spike of glucose in your bloodstream from food as quickly as possible and

b. then have the insulin stop working so that it does not continue to reduce glucose to a point that you have low blood sugar.

Rapid-acting insulin also gives you the flexibility to choose when you want to eat. Because of the fast onset of action, you can give yourself insulin right before you eat, in the middle of your meal, or just after you eat. This is a key factor because if you have to wait longer for insulin to work, such as with a short-acting insulin, you will have to give yourself insulin 30 to 60 minutes *before* you eat; this means you will really have to plan the timing and content of your meals carefully.

Insulin coverage throughout the day is called basal insulin. Basal insulin therapy uses long-acting insulin medications (Lantus or Detemir) that give you coverage throughout the day. This coverage should not have "peaks" or "valleys," but should be relatively the same throughout the day for greatest efficacy. The purpose of this type of dosing is to create insulin levels that are constant throughout the day in order to control glucose produced by the liver.

Intermediate-acting insulin may also be used for basal insulin coverage, but it requires more injections to achieve the desired effect. This is because the duration of action is only about 10 to 16 hours. Intermediate-acting insulin also has a distinct peak which may cause lows. This is not preferred in basal insulin therapy because the goal of this type of therapy is to provide a constant delivery of insulin without peaks or valleys.

Insulin Profiles

Meal-time or Prandial Insulin

Rapid-acting insulins (Lispro, Aspart, Apidra or inhaled insulin) have an onset of action as quickly as 10 to 15 minutes, and its peak action is between 30 to 90 minutes. Rapid-acting insulin only stays effective in the body for three to five hours. So, you can see how fast this insulin starts to work and then leaves the body. Rapid-acting insulin is the fastest working and the shortest duration insulin of all insulins. This makes sense because after digesting food your food is gone and you no longer need insulin.

Short-acting insulin (Humulin R and Novolin R) starts to work in 30 to 60 minutes, peaks in two to three hours, and lasts in the body for five to eight hours. If you use short-acting insulin, you would have to give yourself an injection 30 to 60 minutes before a meal for the insulin to be working at peak effectiveness by the time you eat.

All day insulin coverage or Basal Insulin

Intermediate-acting insulin (NPH insulin) starts to work in two to four hours, its peak action is four to ten hours, and the duration of action is 10 to 16 hours. The duration of intermediate-acting insulin falls short of 24 hours, so two injections are needed to provide all day coverage.

Long-acting insulin (Lantus, Levemir and Tresiba) has the longest duration of action of all the insulins. Long-acting insulins start to work in two to four hours, but studies of Lantus and Tresiba have shown that it does not have any peak action, meaning coverage is consistent throughout the day. The longer duration makes it truly a once-a-day insulin.

(See next page.)

Not a comprehensive drug list

Brand Name	Generic Name	Onset of Action	Peak Effect	Duration of Action
Rapid-acting				
NovoLog	Insulin aspart	10-30 min	30-90 min	3.5 hrs
Humalog	Insulin lispro	10-30 min	30-90 min	3-5 hrs
Apidra	Insulin glulisine	10-30 min	30-90 min	3-5 hrs
Fiasp	Insulin aspart	15 min	60-90 min	5-6 hrs
Tresiba	Insulin inhaled	12 min	35-45 min	1.5-3 hrs
Short-acting				
Humulin R	Insulin Regular	30-60 min	1.5-2 hrs	5-8 hrs
Novolin R	Insulin regular	30-60 min	1.5-2 hrs	5-8 hrs
Intermediate-acting (NPH)				
Humulin N	Insulin NPH	1-2 hrs	4-8 hrs	10-20 hrs
Novolin N	Insulin NPH	1-2 hrs	4-8 hrs	10-20 hrs
Long-acting				
Levemir	Insulin detemir	1 hr	Relatively flat peak	12-20 hrs
Lantus	Insulin glargine	1-2 hrs	No peak	22-24 hrs
Tresiba	Insulin degludec	1-2 hrs	No Peak	Up to 42hr

Prandial Insulin Dosing and the Insulin-to-Carbohydrate Ratio

Glucose is delivered to the body in the form of the carbohydrates you eat. These can be simple or complex carbohydrates, but each is broken down into glucose by your body. Thus, bolus or prandial insulin dosing is directly dependent upon how many grams of carbohydrates you plan to eat at a given meal. Calculating the amount of insulin you should take at mealtime is called the insulin-to-carbohydrate ratio.

Your physician will calculate your insulin-to-carbohydrate ratio using glucose readings performed at home two hours after a meal. Your dosing ratio might look something like this: If your insulin-to-carbohydrate ratio is 1 unit of insulin for every 15 grams of carbohydrates you eat and your meal contains 30 grams of carbohydrates, you should give yourself 2 units of insulin. You will need to adjust your insulin-to-carbohydrate ratio if you are not reaching your goal range.

Correction Factor or Dose Adjustment

To make sure your insulin dosing is correct, it is very important to test your blood glucose before you eat so you can give yourself the right amount. Doing this also allows you to make sure you have enough units of insulin on hand. You may need to adjust the amount of insulin given at mealtime if you are too low or too high prior to your meal. If your pre-meal glucose reading is below 70 mg/dl (or the value that your physician has indicated is low for you), you may need to subtract one or two units from your mealtime insulin so you do not go too low. Conversely, if your glucose is above 180 mg/dl (or the level your physician determined is high for you), you may need to add one or two units to your mealtime insulin. This adjustment is called a Correction Factor or Dose Adjustment. Your physician should develop a Correction Factor or Dose Adjustment Action Plan for you.

In order for you to achieve your blood glucose targets, your Correction Factor Action Plan requires self-monitoring your blood glucose before you eat. In addition, you will need to review a number of questions before you give yourself a bolus or prandial dose of insulin.

Some of these questions are:

- What is my glucose level before I eat? Am I high, low or is my glucose in the target range determined by my doctor?

- If I am high or low, what is my correction factor?

- How many grams of carbohydrates am I going to eat? What is my insulin-to-carbohydrate ratio?

- What am I going to do after I eat? Exercise or rest?

- Is there anything different about this particular meal that may affect my glucose?

Knowing the answer to these questions allows you to make sure you are giving yourself the correct amount of insulin. You can review the questions with your physician so that you feel confident about your correction action plan.

Basal Insulin or Long-Acting Insulin Dosing

Basal insulin is the amount of insulin produced by a

normal pancreas that decreases glucose output from the liver. Long-acting insulins, like Lantus, Tresiba, and Levemir, seek to replicate this insulin secretion rate. They are usually given once a day, at night, and act to stop or slow glucose output from the liver throughout the day. A common method to determine the amount of basal insulin to take at night is to target your insulin dose to achieve a specific range when you take your morning glucose readings. Some physicians use these ranges:

5 to 11 years of age: 70-180 mg/dl

12 years and above: 70-150 mg/dl

Your doctor will help you determine what your normal morning blood glucose range should be and set your insulin dosing accordingly.

Changes in Insulin Dosing

There are situations and activities that can change your glucose levels and affect how much insulin you need to take at a given time. Here are some examples:

- Hot or warm showers change the way insulin works. Warm water increases your blood flow, causing insulin to be absorbed faster. This may cause low blood sugar, so it is not advisable to take a hot shower after administering insulin.

- Exercise changes glucose levels by burning off more glucose. However, glucose utilization in your muscles when you work out is not the same mechanism as insulin-glucose transport. So, if you take insulin and then exercise, glucose utilization and sensitivity are increased, which can lead to hypoglycemia. As a result, the amount of insulin you need is usually reduced. Remember once you take insulin, it cannot be decreased in your body. It not only increases the amount of glucose going into your muscles, but continues to decrease the liver production of glucose, which makes you more susceptible for hypoglycemia.

Therefore, you must test before, during, and after exercise, and adjust your insulin to your tested glucose level. You need to check the timing of your exercise and insulin shot before exercise, because your body will be more sensitive to insulin after activity. Also, your muscles are still metabolically active long after you stop exercising and the increased insulin sensitivity will promote glucose uptake. Any lows you experience from exercising can happen hours after you have ended your activity.

- Growth and sex hormones will change glucose levels and insulin dosing will need to be adjusted. During the teen years, diabetes control may be more difficult and may require more insulin as growth and sex hormones become more prevalent in the body. These hormones make it more difficult for insulin to work, but the condition should reverse after puberty.

- Stress and illness change glucose levels and you need to watch your insulin dosing closely at these times. During periods of stress or illness, glucose levels are very hard to control. Therefore, the more you test your glucose levels, the better you can control your diabetes.

These are not the only circumstances that can affect your insulin dosing, but are the most common. The best course is to check your glucose levels frequently and carefully monitor your dosing.

Injecting Insulin

Working with your physician to determine your bolus and basal insulin dosing is the first step in learning to use insulin as an effective tool in diabetes control. The second step is knowing how to administer and store your insulin so that you maximize its effectiveness.

You will want to make sure you rotate through different sites for your insulin injections to prevent swelling of the skin, hard lumps, or the development of fat deposits. If swelling does occur, do not use that injection site until the swelling is gone; these changes will alter your skin's ability to absorb insulin. Do not inject close to your belly button, or near moles or scars, as tissue there is tougher and insulin absorption will not be as consistent. If you inject in your upper arm, only use the outer back area where there is more fat. It can be hard to pinch your upper arm when you are injecting yourself, so try pressing your upper arm against a wall or door. If you inject in your thighs, stay away from your inner thighs; if your thighs rub together when you walk, it might make the injection site sore. Do not inject in an area that will be exercised soon. Exercising increases blood flow, which causes long-acting insulin to be absorbed at a rate that is faster than you need. Insulin is absorbed at different speeds depending on where you inject.

According to Eli Lilly and Company, the leading manufacturer of insulin, insulin enters the blood:

- Fastest from the abdomen (stomach)
- A little slower from the arms
- Even slower from the legs
- Slowest from the buttocks

Talk to your physician about using all these sites and see if there could be any concerns.

Storing Insulin

Storing your insulin properly is important. All unopened insulin should be stored in the refrigerator at a temperature of 36°to 46°F (2° to 8°C). Insulin manufacturers advise that most open insulin vials kept at room temperature are only good for 28 days and should be thrown out after this to avoid the risk of bacterial growth. If you keep an open vial in the refrigerator, you still have to throw it out after 28 days. Unopened insulin kept in the refrigerator will be good until the expiration date. The expiration date is found on the top of the box the insulin came in; instructions for storing your insulin can be found inside the box.

Insulin is made up of amino acids, which are sensitive to temperature extremes. This means that you should not use any insulin that has been frozen or exposed to excessive heat or sunlight, because these extreme temperatures can destroy the insulin.

You may keep your current open insulin bottle in the refrigerator or at room temperature. If you keep it in the refrigerator, it is best to warm it to room temperature before you give yourself a shot. Doing so will help make the injection less painful and less likely to sting or to cause red spots.

Glucagon

Glucagon is an injection used in emergencies, such as unconsciousness, when your blood glucose level is so low that raising it quickly is necessary. If you are unconscious, an injection is preferred because there is a risk that your airway may become blocked if anything is administered orally (by mouth).

Everyone who is insulin dependent should have a glucagon injection kit, but your physician will advise if a glucagon kit is appropriate for you. Ask your physician to show you how to use the kit, and work with you and your family to develop and review your emergency action plan. In addition, when you pick up your kit at the pharmacy, make sure to ask the pharmacist to show you how to use the injector. Remember, an emergency is not the time to learn how to use the glucagon kit.

It is important to place your kit in a specific location in your house and tell all your family members where it is in case of an emergency. You may also want to have a kit at work, and make sure your coworkers understand when and how to help you. An action plan for administering glucagon is a **must**. Go over your action plan and rehearse it once or twice with your whole family.

Summary

The amazing discovery of insulin has stopped a once fatal disease and has allowed insulin-dependent people to live full and healthy lives. With the development of rapid-acting and long-acting insulin, people with insulin-dependent diabetes can come much closer to simulating the natural secretion of insulin from the pancreas.

Because ultimate responsibility for your health lies only with you, it is vital that you take the time to learn about and understand your insulin dosing, monitor your glucose frequently around meals and exercise, and know how to properly store and administer your insulin.

Exciting research on diabetes continues. I have the privilege of working as a Research Information Volunteer with the Juvenile Diabetes Research Foundation. Our meetings include scientists from all over the world who are working not only on better control of diabetes, but also on a cure. While that may still be some time off, it is so encouraging to know that many of the brightest minds in medicine are working to make life with diabetes as manageable as possible.

ABOUT THE AUTHOR

Christine Schaffer received her Doctor of Pharmacy from the University of the Pacific School of Pharmacy in Stockton, California, and was granted a Bachelor of Science in Clinical Laboratory Science from the University of Nevada, Reno. She is licensed in Florida, California, and Nevada State Boards of Pharmacy. She is also a Board-Certified Pharmacotherapy Specialist and Board Certified Florida Pharmacist Consultant as well as a licensed Clinical Laboratory Scientist.

Dr. Schaffer is the co-founder and Chief Clinical Officer of American Health Care, a health management company that specializes in delivering patient-centric pharmacy benefit, population health and therapy management programs that emphasize clinical excellence. She is also the developer of a proprietary software system that provides virtual clinical records used by hospitals across the country. She is the preceptor for the company's pharmacy residency program and co-founded the United American Pharmacy Network. She has been affiliated with the American College of Managed Care Pharmacy, the American College of Clinical Pharmacy, the American Society of Health System Pharmacists, and the Academy of Managed Care Pharmacy.

When not at work, Dr. Schaffer enjoys the company of her family, has a black belt in Taekwondo, loves to ski, weight lift, and hike. She is an avid supporter of the Juvenile Diabetes Research Association and has served on the Juvenile Diabetes Research foundation board for 7 years. Dr. Schaffer has also served in board meetings of several consulting companies, as well as human rights advocacy groups for the mentally disabled.

Glossary

A	
ADA	American Diabetes Association
Adipose	Tissue made up mainly of fat cells
Adipocytes	Fat cells
Aerobic	Literally "requiring air;" refers to activities that affect large muscle groups that require the lungs to work harder, such as walking, running, cycling, etc.
Afferent arterioles	Arteries going into the kidneys
Albumin; albuminuria	A protein made by the liver; the presence of albumin in urine
Aldosterone	Aldosterone regulates sodium and potassium levels, helping to maintain both blood pressure and bodily fluids.
Alpha cells	Cells found in the pancreas; they synthesize and secrete glucagon
Atherosclerosis	Literally "hard paste;" a condition where fatty material collects along the walls of arteries; it may harden and form plaques and eventually block arteries
Autoimmune response	When the body creates antibodies that kill off the body's own cells; a condition where the immune system mistakenly attacks and destroys healthy body tissue
B	
Baroreceptor	A mechanism that detects the pressure of fluid flowing through a vessel, such as blood through a blood vessel
Basal insulin secretion	The amount of insulin needed to maintain blood glucose levels at a steady state during overnight and between meal periods
Body Mass Index (BMI)	A number calculated from your height and weight that is a fairly reliable indicator of body fat
C	
Cardiovascular	The circulatory system comprising the heart and blood vessels which carry nutrients and oxygen to the tissues of the body
Catecholamines	Hormones produced by the adrenal glands in times of physical or emotional stress; the major ones are dopamine, norepinephrine, and epinephrine
Chylomicron	A lipoprotein produced by the small intestine to transport fat

D	
Distal tubule	Found inside the kidneys; carries filtered fluid away from the kidneys in the formation of urine. It regulates potassium, sodium, calcium, and pH
Diuretic	Any drug that promotes the formation of urine by the kidneys; helps shed excess water in the system
DM	Diabetes mellitus
Duration of action	The length of time insulin still has some effect in the body
E	
Edema	Fluid accumulation beneath the skin
Exogenous	An action or object coming from outside the body
F	
Fasting blood glucose test	A blood test performed after at least eight hours without food or drink (except water)
G	
Gastroparesis	A condition that affects the ability of the stomach to empty its contents
Glomerular	Pertaining to the glomerulus, a tiny structure in the kidney that filters blood to form urine
Glomerular filtration rate (GFR)	An estimate done to assess the severity of nephropathy or kidney disease
Glucose	A type of sugar the body uses for energy
Glucose post glucose challenge test	A test in which you are given a 75-gram glucose drink and blood glucose is tested two hours later
Glycogen	The form in which glucose is stored in the body for later use
Glucagon	A hormone secreted by the pancreas that raises blood sugar levels
H	
HDL	High density lipoprotein, good cholesterol, helps eliminate cholesterol from the bloodstream
Hepatic	Having to do with the liver
Hyperglycemia	High blood sugar; excessive amounts of glucose in the blood
Hyperinsulinemia	Excess levels of insulin in the blood
Hypertension	The medical term for blood pressure that is above normal. A blood pressure reading of greater than 130/80 for people with diabetes is considered hypertension
Hypoglycemia	Low blood sugar; too little glucose in the blood
Hypoxia	Lack of adequate oxygen supply

I	
Impaired fasting glucose (IFG)	The glucose results of a fasting blood test that fall between normal glucose levels and diabetes
Impaired glucose tolerance (IGT)	A two-hour test result after drinking 75 grams of glucose that falls between normal glucose levels and diabetes
Insulin	A hormone that promotes the absorption of glucose into cells
Insulin resistance	A condition in which the body produces insulin but cannot use it properly
Ischemia	Decreased blood flow resulting in little or no oxygen delivery to tissues and organs
J	
Juxtaglomerular cells	Cells located in the afferent arterioles of the kidneys that synthesize, store, and secrete renin
K	
Ketoacidosis	When the body uses fat for energy because it cannot use glucose due to low or no insulin resulting in a buildup of ketones
L	
LDL	Low density lipoprotein, "bad cholesterol," carries cholesterol and other fats to various parts of the body
Lipolysis	The breakdown of fats
Lipoprotein lipase (LPL)	An enzyme that breaks down fat
M	
Macroalbuminuria	A condition characterized by especially high levels of a protein, albumin, being leaked into the urine
Macrovascular	Pertaining to the larger blood vessels
Mechanism of action	The way a drug works in the body; the pathway it takes to achieve the intended results
Microalbuminuria	A condition where the kidneys leak small amounts of a protein, albumin, into the urine
Microvascular	Having to do with very small branches of arteries
mg/dl	Milligrams per deciliter, a test measurement unit
mmol/l	millimoles per liter; millimole is a unit of molecular weight
mmHg	milligrams of mercury; unit of measurement for blood pressure readings

N	
Nephrons	A structural unit of the kidneys, mainly involved with regulating fluid concentrations by filtering the blood, reabsorbing what is needed, and excreting the rest
Nephropathy	Kidney disease
Neuropathy	Nerve disease
O	
Onset of action	The length of time it takes for insulin to start to work
P	
Pancreas	An organ just below the stomach that creates and secretes insulin into the bloodstream
Peak action	The length of time insulin is most effective
Peripheral arterial disease	Narrowing of the arteries, mostly in the lower part of the body
Polydipsia	Excessive thirst; thirsty all the time
Polyphagia	Excessive hunger; hungry all the time
Polyuria	Excessive urination
Postprandial	After eating
Pressor	Relating to or producing an increase in blood pressure
Q	
R	
Reabsorption	The process of something being absorbed again
	Changes to the size, shape, or function of the heart after injury to the ventricles, stemming from hypertension, myocardial infarction, congestive heart failure or other conditions
Renal	Having to do with the kidneys
Renin	A protein released by the kidneys that causes vasoconstriction
S	
Secretagogue	A substance that causes another substance to be secreted
Silent Ischemia	Small artery blockages with no symptoms of chest pain
U	

V	
Vasoconstriction	Narrowing of the blood vessels from contraction of the surrounding muscle wall of the vessels
Vasodilatation; vasodilator	Widening of the blood vessels from relaxing of the surrounding muscle wall; an agent that opens or widens blood vessels by relaxing their muscular walls
Vasopressin	A hormone secreted by the pituitary gland that acts on the kidneys and blood vessels to help reabsorb water in the body
Visceral fat; visceral adipose tissue	Fat located with the abdomen surrounding the visceral organs, i.e., the heart, lungs, intestines, liver, kidneys, pancreas, and spleen
W, X, Y, Z	

Bibliography

NCHS Data Brief ▪ No. 492 ▪ March 2024 U.S. Department Of Health And Human Services Centers for Disease Control and Prevention National Center for Health Statistics, "Mortality in the United States," 2022 Kenneth D. Kochanek, M.A., Sherry L. Murphy, B.S., Jiaquan Xu, M.D., and Elizabeth Arias, Ph.D

Number of people with diabetes increases to 38.4 million. May 15, 2024.

Centers for Disease Control and Prevention. National Diabetes Statistics Report website. https://www.cdc.gov/diabetes/data/statistics-report/in dex.html. Accessed August 19, 2024.

American Diabetes Association. Diabetes Care 2023; Volume 46 (Suppl.1), Standards of Diabetes Care, January 2023.

American Diabetes Association Professional Practice Committee; 16. Diabetes Care in the Hospital: Standards of Medical Care in Diabetes—2022. Diabetes Care 1 January 2022; 45 (Supplement_1): S244–S253

USAFACTS, October 6, 2023 by Usa Facts Team. Usafacts.org.

2023 national diabetes fact sheet: diagnosed and undiagnosed diabetes in the United States, all ages. U.S. Department of Health and Human Services, Centers for Disease Control and Prevention.

American Diabetes Association. "Standards of medical care in diabetes – 2022," Diabetes Care 33, suppl. 1, January 2022.

Amiel, S.A. 2009. "Hypoglycemia in patients with type 1 diabetes." Therapy for diabetes mellitus and related disorder, ed., H.E. Lebovitz, Alexandria, VA: American Diabetes Association.

Bakris, G., M. Williams, L. Dworkin, W. Elliott, M. Epstein,

R. Toto, et al.. 2000. "Preserving Renal Function in Adults With Hypertension and Diabetes: A Consensus Approach," American Journal of Kidney Diseases , 36 (3), 646-661.

Bek, T. 2000. "Histopathology and pathophysiology of diabetic retinopathy." Diabetic Retinopathy, ed. van Bijsterveld, O.P., London: Martin Dunitz, Ltd.:169-187.

Biaggioni, I. 2009. "Postural hypotension," Therapy for diabetes mellitus and related disorder, ed. H.E. Lebovitiz, Alexandria, VA: American Diabetes Association.

Boulton, A. 2009. "Painful or insensitive lower extremity," Therapy for diabetes mellitus and related disorders, ed. H.E. Lebovitiz, Alexandria, VA: American Diabetes Association.

Chen, H.C. 2005. "Classification and diagnosis of diabetic retinopathy," Vascular complications of diabetes: current issues in pathogenesis and treatment. ed. R. Donnelly, E.S. Horton, Malden, MA: Blackwell Publishing Ltd., 139-150.

Chobanian, A., G. Bakris, H. Black, W. Cushman, L. Green, J. Izzo, et al. 2003. "The Seventh Report of the Joint National Committee on Prevention, Detection, Evaluation, and Treatment of High Blood Pressure: The JNC 7 Report," Journal of the American Medical Association, 2561-2572.

Critchley, J., S. Capewell. 2010. "Mortality risk reduction associated with smoking cessation in patients with coronary heart disease: a systematic review," Journal of the American Medical Association, 2003; 290(1):86-97.

Davis, A., I. Duka, G. Bakris. 2009. "Diabetic Nephropathy," Therapy for diabetes mellitus and related disorders, ed. H.E. Lebovitiz, Alexandria, VA: American Diabetes Association.

Browning, D.J., Glassman, A.R., et al. 2007. "Relationship between optical coherence tomography-measured central retinal thickness and visual acuity in diabetic macular edema," Ophthalmology, 114:525-536.

Diabetic Retinopathy Research Group. 1976. "Preliminary report on effects of photocoagulation therapy," American Journal of Ophthalmology. 81: 383-396.

DiPiro, J., R. Talbert, G. Yee, G. Matzke, B. Wells, L. Posey. 2005. Pharmacotherapy: A pathophysiologic approach. New York: McGraw-Hill.

Duka, I, G. Bakris. 2009. "Treatment-associated renal dysfunction in patients with diabetes," Therapy for diabetes mellitus and related disorders, ed. H.E. Lebovitiz, Alexandria, VA: American Diabetes Association.

Framingham Heart Study. Retrieved from www.framing-hamheartstudy.org

Andersson, C., Johnson, A.D., Benjamin, E.J. et al. 70-year legacy of the Framingham Heart Study. Nat Rev Cardiol 16, 687–698 (2019). https://doi.org/10.1038/s41569-019-0202-5

Friedman, E. 2009. "Chronic kidney disease," Therapy for diabetes mellitus and related disorders, ed. H.E. Lebovitiz, Alexandria, VA: American Diabetes Association

Funnell, M. M., R.M. Anderson. 2009. "Role of diabetes education in patient management," Therapy for diabetes mellitus and related disorders, ed. H.E. Lebovitiz, Alexandria, VA: American Diabetes Association.

Garrett, R., C. Grisham. 1995. Biochemistry. University of Virginia: Saunders College Publishing.

Greenhouse, L., C.K. Lardinois. 1996. "Alcohol-associated diabetes mellitus. A review of the impact of alcohol consumption on carbohydrate metabolism," Archives of Family Medicine. Vol. 5.

Horton, E.S. 2009. "Exercise," Therapy for diabetes mellitus and related disorders, ed. H.E. Lebovitiz, Alexandria, VA: American Diabetes Association.

Klein, R., B.E.K. Klein, S.E. Moss, et al. 1998. "The Wisconsin Epidemiologic Study of Diabetic Retinopathy: SVII. The 14-year incidence and progression of diabetic retinopathy and associated risk factors in type 1 diabetes," Ophthalmology,105; 1801-1815.

Kurra, S., H. Ginsberg. 2009. "Diabetic dyslipidemia," Therapy for diabetes mellitus and related disorders, ed. H.E. Lebovitiz, Alexandria, VA: American Diabetes Association.

Massachusetts Medical Society. 1993. "The effect of intensive treatment of diabetes on the development and progression of long-term complications in-dependent diabetes mellitus," The New England Journal of Medicine, Vol. 329, No 14.

Mayo Clinic Proceedings. 2006. "Consensus guidelines: assessment, diagnosis, and treatment of diabetic peripheral neuropathic pain," April, vol. 81, no. 4.

Miller, D., P.C. Magnante. 2004. "Optics of the normal eye," Ophthalmology – 2nd ed, ed. M. Yanoff, M., J.S. Duker, St. Louis, Missouri: Mosby; 59-67.

Morello, C.M. 2007. "Etiology and natural history of diabetic retinopathy: an overview," American Journal of Health-System Pharmacy, 64, Supp. 12.

Mulvaney, Michael J. 2002. "Small artery remodeling and significance in the development of hypertension," News in Physiological Sciences Vol. 17, No 3, 105-109.

New England Journal of Medicine. 2005. Intensive Diabetes Treatment and Cardiovascular Disease in Patients with Type 1 Diabetes: The Diabetes Control and Complications Trial/ Epidemiology of Diabetes Interventions and Complications (DCCT/EDIC) Study Research Group.

Vol. 353, No. 25.

Resnicoff, S., D. Pascolini, D. Etya'ale. 2004. "Global data on visual impairment in the year 2002," Bulletin of World Health Organization, 82:844-851.

Rosenblatt, B.J., W.E. Benson. 2004. "Diabetic retinopathy," ed. Yanoff M., Duker J.S., Ophthalmology, 2nd ed. St. Louis, Missouri: Mosby; 877-886.

Rosendorff, C., H. Black, B. Gersh, J. Gore, J.J. Izzo, et al. 2007. "Treatment of Hypertension in the Prevention and management of Ischemic Heart Disease," Circulation: A Journal of the American Heart Association, 2761-2788.

Zemel, Michael B. 1995. "Insulin resistance, obesity and hypertension: an overview," The Journal of Nutrition, American Institute of Nutrition, 125: 1715S-1717S.

Barrett-Connor E, Wingard D, Wong N, Goldberg R. Chapter 18: Heart disease and diabetes (PDF, 1.07 MB). In: Cowie CC, Casagrande SS, Menke A, et al, eds. Diabetes in America, 3rd ed. NIH Pub No. 17-1468. National Institutes of Health; 2018:18.1–18.30

Pikula A, Howard BV, Seshadri S. Chapter 19: Stroke and diabetes (PDF, 493.93 KB). In: Cowie CC, Casagrande SS, Menke A, et al, eds. Diabetes in America, 3rd ed. NIH Pub No. 17-1468. National Institutes of Health; 2018:19.1–19.23

Centers for Disease Control and Prevention. National Diabetes Statistics Report website. https://www.cdc.gov/diabetes/data/statistics-report/ind ex.html. Accessed [10/22/2022].

Whelton PK, Carey RM, Aronow WS, Casey DE, Collins KJ, Dennison Himmelfarb C, DePalma SM, Gidding S, Jamerson KA, Jones DW, et al.. 2017 ACC/AHA/AAPA/ABC/ACPM/AGS/APhA/ASH/A

SPC/NMA/PCNA guideline for the prevention, detection, evaluation, and management of high blood pressure in adults: a report of the American College of Cardiology/American Heart Association Task Force on clinical practice guidelines. Hypertension. 2018; 71:e13–e115.

Aspirin Use to Prevent Cardiovascular Disease: Preventive Medication. U.S. Preventative Task force. https://www.uspreventiveservicestaskforce.org/uspstf/recommendation/aspirin-to-prevent-cardiovascular-disease-preventive-medication. Accessed November 2022.

www.ingramcontent.com/pod-product-compliance
Lightning Source LLC
Chambersburg PA
CBHW062218270326
41930CB00009B/1781

9 798990 014312